Hear What You've Been Missing

HOW TO COPE WITH
HEARING LOSS

QUESTIONS
ANSWERS
OPTIONS

DONNA S. WAYNER, Ph.D.

CHRONIMED PUBLISHING

Hear What You've Been Missing: How to Cope with
Hearing Loss © 1998 by Donna S. Wayner

Library of Congress Cataloging-in-Publication Data
Wayner, Donna S.
Hear what you've been missing / by Donna S. Wayner

     p.   cm.

Includes index.

ISBN 1-56561-148-9; $14.95

Edited by: Renée Nicholls
Cover Design: Pear Design
Text Design & Production: David Enyeart
Art/Production Manager: Claire Lewis
Printed in the United States

Published by
Chronimed Publishing
P.O. Box 59032
Minneapolis, MN 55459-0032

10   9   8   7   6   5   4   3   2   1

Notice: Consult a Health Care Professional.
Because individual cases and needs vary, readers are advised
to seek the guidance of a licensed physician, registered
dietitian, or other health care professional before making
changes in their health care regimen. This book is intended
for informational purposes only and is not for use as an
alternative to appropriate medical care. While every effort
has been made to ensure that the information is the most
current available, new research findings, being released
with increasing frequency, may invalidate some data.

For Mary Bass Shpikula and Vera Spikula, who as role-models and teachers provided guidance and inspiration and taught me to listen to the beauty of the hours.

14 *95*

1. What Is Hearing Loss?

2. How Does Hearing Loss Affect Daily Life?

3. Is Hearing Loss Common?

4. What Are Signs of Hearing Loss in Adults?

5. What Are Warning Signs of Hearing Loss in Children?

6. What Do I Do if My Child or I Seem to Have Lost Some Hearing?

7. How Is Hearing Tested?

8. How Do I Read My Audiogram?

9. How Does My Hearing Test Differ from the Tests of Others?

10. How Is Hearing Loss Described?

11. Are There Different Types of Hearing Loss?

12. How Does the Ear Work?

13. Do Many People Have Head Noises?

14. How Can I Be Hard of Hearing and Yet Be Painfully Sensitive to Noise?

15. How Are Dizziness and Hearing Loss Related?

16. Can Hearing Loss Affect the Voice and the Way People Speak?

17. How Can I Explain My Hearing Loss to Others?

CONTENTS

Figures

Acknowledgments

IT'S SUNG IN *The Sound of Music*, "Nothing comes from nothing," which is so true for this book. It has emerged from the expressed needs of many friends and patients. Their frequently asked questions formed the basis for the included information.

I am grateful to those who contributed directly to the completion of this project, especially Virginia H. Conard, who skillfully prepared the figures. Most particularly, I am sincerely appreciative of the support and patient encouragement given daily by Peter, my husband.

Preface

MANY PEOPLE MAY still feel that hearing loss is something to be hidden and not talked about. Much misunderstanding exists. Fortunately, this attitude is changing, and it is hoped that this book, designed to provide an overview of nontechnical information to answer those questions you may have about hearing loss, will help bring about this change. The more that is realized about hearing loss in general and about the many specific helps available to overcome the effects of hearing loss, the fewer the number of people who will suffer isolation and misunderstanding because of an impaired hearing mechanism.

Many tools and strategies are available to assist people who don't hear well. These, plus the causes of hearing loss and a list of resources for help for yourself or someone you care about, are covered in this book.

Much can be done to remedy the frustrations and confusions brought about by impaired hearing. Take the step to better communication. If you or someone you care about cannot hear well, read on.

Hear What You've
Been Missing

CHAPTER ONE

Hearing Loss

1. What Is Hearing Loss?

A hearing loss is defined as a reduction in a person's ability to hear. To avoid any confusion over the terms used to describe reduced hearing, throughout this book the general term *hearing loss* will be used to include all degrees of hearing impairment however great or small. But having a hearing loss means more than simply not being able to hear well. A wide range of experiences are linked to our ability to hear, and a wide range of problems may be associated with hearing loss. Hearing loss is invisible and, because of that, often ignored. But it is very real. A hearing loss can affect every aspect of our daily lives.

2. How Does Hearing Loss Affect Daily Life?

Our hearing ability keeps us connected to the world. We know what is going on just by monitoring the surroundings with our ears. Hearing helps to keep us safe in traffic and on the job. If we cannot hear well, then it might be harder to use the telephone or watch television without turning up the volume. We may not always hear the doorbell or telephone when it rings. We may be able to hear some people better than others, depending on how well they articulate or if their voice is low- or high-pitched. At work or in school, hearing loss makes it harder to hear important information.

Without good hearing, it is also harder to communicate, and this loss can cause psychological and social difficulties. Just about everything we do in life is based on verbal communication. If we have difficulty hearing, our ability to talk with others is changed. We cannot exchange our thoughts and feelings spontaneously. Hearing loss can affect how clearly people speak since they may hear their own voice sounds in a distorted way. Repeated instances of unheard or incorrectly heard communications are frustrating for the individual with a hearing loss as well as for those who are attempting to converse. This may result in fewer attempts to communicate. Family and social relationships can be affected.

Hearing loss may limit a person's ability to enjoy many forms of entertainment, such as television, music, radio, and theater. This also results in withdrawal and social isolation. Access to information normally available through personal communication and the media is limited.

Hearing is a 360-degree sense, grounding us to the world and connecting us to the environment. Hearing loss limits this connectedness.

3. Is Hearing Loss Common?

It is estimated that as many as 28 million people, one in ten in the United States, suffer some degree of hearing loss. As with the other senses, hearing tends to deteriorate as we get older. By age sixty-five, more than one-third of the American population is affected by hearing loss. Fortunately, many of these people have only a slight degree of loss causing difficulties only in certain life situations. Others have more severe hearing losses or profound loss.

However, hearing loss in not limited to the elderly. It is experienced by people of all ages. Some have experienced hearing loss since birth; others experience it later in life.

The proportion of people with a hearing disorder is increasing because current medical care can save more high-risk infants than ever before; some of these infants will have hearing disorders. Also, more of us are being exposed to extremely loud noises on the job or in our recreation. In addition, we are living longer and reaching the ages when impaired hearing becomes more common.

Hearing loss is the most common handicapping condition, and yet it is the least understood. It is important to realize that help is available for every degree of hearing loss. Chapter 4 deals with different types of hearing aids, their benefits, and their limitations. It will review how to get a hearing aid and learn to hear again with amplification. Assistive devices, supplementary aids for daily living, will be discussed in Chapter 5. Various strategies and techniques for creative coping with some of the difficulties resulting from hearing loss will be addressed in Chapter 6.

There is always something that can be done to minimize the problems we face: the most serious problem is doing nothing at all.

4. What Are Signs of Hearing Loss in Adults?

If you have a hearing loss, sounds may seem loud enough, but not clear. People may seem to be mumbling or talking too quickly. Quiet sounds, such as a clock ticking, birds singing, or voices from another room, just cannot be heard as well as before. You may hear some people's voices better than others. You may find that facing the speaker helps you to hear better. It is difficult to understand what is being said in a group when there is any background noise. Group conversations are more and more difficult to follow. You might find that meetings, groups, parties, and movies are not as rewarding as before. It is harder to keep up with small talk. You may favor one ear over the other. You need to ask for things to be repeated. Sometimes, you misunderstand what has been said. Others may tell you that you have the radio or television turned up "too loud" or that you speak too loudly or too softly. You may be startled when someone enters the room. You may have difficulty locating the source or direction of sounds. Loud sounds may seem more sharp and annoying than before. You may hear ringing or buzzing in your ears. Read through the following checklist. If you answer yes to more than five of the signs and symptoms listed, see your physician *(see Question 6 in this chapter)*.

COMMON SIGNS AND SYMPTOMS OF HEARING LOSS

Do you...
frequently have to ask for repetition?
have trouble hearing when you are spoken to from another room?
feel that you hear sound but do not understand speech clearly?
feel that people are mumbling?
have trouble hearing when there is noise around you?
need to turn the radio or TV volume up loud to hear well?
have difficulty hearing women's or children's voices?
have to turn one ear toward the person speaking?
have trouble hearing when you can't see the speaker's face?
need to be close to the person speaking?
become anxious or tired in social situations because you cannot understand what is being said?
have to strain to hear?
frequently misunderstand what is said?
have ringing or buzzing in your ear(s)?

Do others tell you that you...
do not react to loud sounds?
do not respond when spoken to?
turn the radio or TV volume up too high?
speak loudly or shout in conversation?
are missing what is being said?
do not hear sounds coming from behind you?
have had a change in your speech?

5. What Are Warning Signs of Hearing Loss in Children?

Some general warning signs include the following:

- The child seems to respond inconsistently to sound, sometimes hearing and sometimes not.

- The child intently watches the speaker's face.

- The child often says "What?" when spoken to.

- The child exhibits behaviors that seem to favor one ear, such as tilting the head to the left or right when listening.

- There is a history of hearing loss in the family.

- The child's mother had rubella (German measles) during pregnancy *(see Question 2 in Chapter 2)*.

- There is a history of blood incompatibility or difficulty in pregnancy.

- The child has had frequent high fevers.

- The child has a history of chronic ear infections.

- The child frequently complains of hurting ears.

- The child seems to respond better to low- or high-pitched sounds.

- There is a change in how loudly or how much the child babbles or talks.

If you suspect a hearing loss, examine the child's speech and language development. The speech of children who have a hearing loss may sound different or less clear because they will be imitating a distorted signal.

Many children have had a hearing impairment since birth and have therefore not heard speech and language of the same quality and quantity as that experienced by children with normal hearing. As a result, their language acquisition is an ongoing, effort-filled sequence instead of a gradual, easy, natural process. Consider the scores of times small children hear a word before they can learn to actually say it. Children with a hearing loss do not hear as many words in their surroundings as easily, and consequently they may build a vocabulary at a much slower pace. Their words may also be missing word endings (e.g., *s, ing*), and short words (e.g., *the, is, it*) may be missing from their speech. The children's written work may also reflect their inability to hear.

These specific age-related behaviors can signal a hearing loss in infants and toddlers:

BEFORE SIX MONTHS

- The child doesn't startle in some way, such as a blink of the eyes or a jerk of the body or a change of activity in response to sudden, loud sounds.

- The child doesn't imitate sounds such as cooing or babbling.

- The child shows no response to noise-making toys.

- The child doesn't respond to or is not soothed by the sound of her mother's voice.

BY SIX MONTHS

- The child doesn't search for sounds by shifting eyes or turning the head from side to side.

BY TEN MONTHS

- The child doesn't show some kind of response to his name.

- He reduces his amount of vocal behaviors, such as babbling.

BY TWELVE MONTHS

- The child shows no response to common household sounds, such as pots banging, running water, or footsteps from behind.

- The child yells when imitating sounds.

- The child doesn't respond to someone's voice by turning her head or body in all directions to search for the source.

BY FIFTEEN MONTHS

- The child isn't beginning to imitate many sounds or isn't attempting to say simple words.

- In order to get the child's attention, you consistently have to raise your voice.

6. What Do I Do if My Child or I Seem to Have Lost Some Hearing?

If you suspect that your child has a hearing loss or if you feel that sounds are not as loud as you need them to be, or that speech is muffled, it is a good idea to first have your family physician check for wax in the ear canals, infection, or a treatable disease. If the problem can be treated medically or surgically, pursue that treatment. If this is not possible, or if after treatment you or your child still has some difficulty hearing, investigate hearing help with an audiologist. To begin, ask your physician for a signed statement or form called a "medical clearance" saying that the hearing loss has been medically evaluated and that you or your child may be considered a candidate for hearing aids. This form is required by law before a hearing aid dispenser can provide you with a hearing aid. (Adults over eighteen may sign a waiver of this regulation, but for your best hearing health you should obtain a medical checkup instead.)

Then arrange for a hearing test to determine how much hearing loss there is. Get a complete hearing evaluation from a licensed audiologist who is a Fellow in the American Academy of Audiology (FAAA) and/or one with a Certificate of Clinical Competence in Audiology (CCC-A) issued by the American Speech Language and Hearing Association (ASHA). Do not confuse the FAAA or CCC-A certification with the description used by many hearing aid dealers of "Board Certified," which is granted by the National Hearing Aid Society (NHAS). NHAS is a trade association of hearing aid dealers.

Audiologists can measure hearing ability and identify the degree of loss. They can design and direct a rehabilitation program, recommend and fit the most appropriate hearing aids, and measure the hearing improvement from the use of hearing aids. They will provide guidance and training on how to use the new hearing aids and recommend the use of other assistive technology if appropriate. They can also teach speechreading. They can help you or your child to find solutions that reduce the effects of hearing loss by working with your spouse, family, employer, teacher, caregiver, or other medical specialists. In addition, audiologists evaluate balance, vertigo and dizziness disorders.

If a hearing aid is recommended, be certain to arrange for a trial of at least thirty days through a facility that will assist you or your child in becoming oriented to the new experience of hearing with amplification. Remember, it is a learning experience that does require time, practice, and patience. *Much more will be described about hearing aids and an adjustment program to their use in Chapter 4.*

7. How Is Hearing Tested?

Hearing tests are given as outpatient services in local hospitals, by audiologists in private practice, or in association with otologists or otolaryngologists. People of all ages can be tested, from newborn infants to aging adults. There is a wide range of hearing tests. Some are quite complicated and used in special diagnostic circumstances; a simple test of hearing ability, called *pure tone audiometry*, takes only a few minutes. For the simple test, you are asked to listen to a series of tones, each of a different pitch (frequency), which are presented as short bursts of sound, first to one ear and then to the other. Usually, the tones are heard through headphones and repeated with a small vibrator placed behind the ear. The loudness (intensity) of each tone is gradually reduced until you can just barely hear that it is still there. This is called your *threshold of hearing* and is marked on a chart called an *audiogram*. As the threshold for each tone is charted, a picture results, indicating the range of sounds you can hear. Red circles are used to chart the results of your test for the right ear, and a blue *X* is used to record your responses when sounds are heard in the left ear.

The completed audiogram represents a person's hearing ability. It shows how intense sound needs to be before you can hear it, and it also shows how loud certain pitches of sounds or frequencies need to be before you can hear them. It is important to know how well you hear the frequencies that make up the sounds of speech.

In addition to the test for pure tones, you will be given a test in which you listen to lists of selected words or sentences that you must repeat. This test measures how well you recognize words and can show how well you understand conversation. It is called *speech audiometry.*

8. How Do I Read My Audiogram?

An audiogram is a drawing that charts your responses to the sounds presented during a hearing test *(see Figure 1-1)*. The markings on the graph show how loud differently pitched sounds need to be before you can hear them. The pitched sounds or frequencies are charted across the top of the graph from a low frequency, 125 Hertz, to high frequency, 8000 Hertz. *Hertz* denotes the pitch or frequency of sound in cycles per second and

FIGURE 1-1

THE AUDIOGRAM

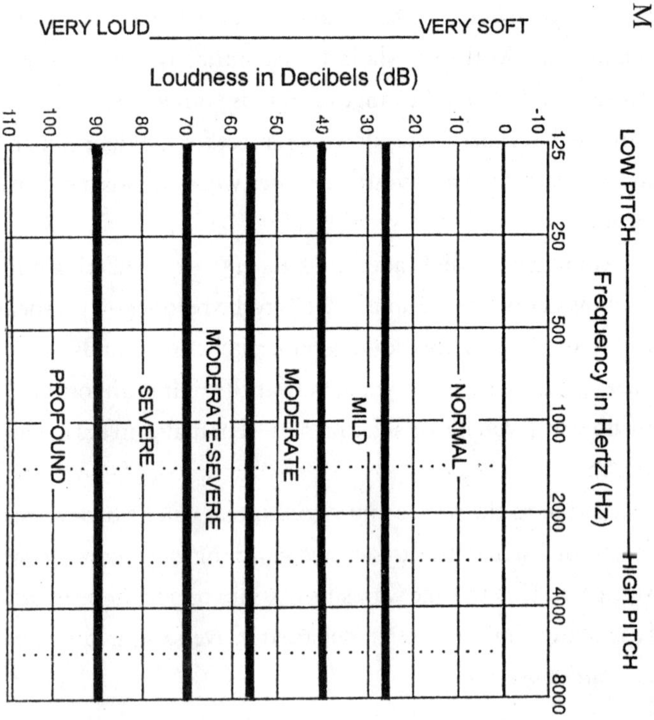

VERY LOUD_____VERY SOFT

Loudness in Decibels (dB)

	125	250	500	1000	2000	4000	8000
-10							
0							
10				NORMAL			
20							
30				MILD			
40				MODERATE			
50							
60				MODERATE-SEVERE			
70							
80				SEVERE			
90							
100				PROFOUND			
110							

LOW PITCH————— Frequency in Hertz (Hz) —————HIGH PITCH

is abbreviated *Hz*. The frequencies (or different pitches) measured include 250 and 500 Hz, which are low frequencies; 1000 and 2000 Hz, which are pitched in the middle range, and 4000 through 8000 Hz, which are high frequencies. Like a piano keyboard, the lower tones are on the left side, and as you move to the right on the graph, the pitch of the sounds gets higher.

The measurements that run vertically on the left side of the audiogram represent the loudness level. The loudness of the sounds is measured in decibels (abbreviated *dB*).

Sounds are softest to the human ear at the top of the audiogram, near 0 dB. 0 dB is the softest level that people with normal hearing can detect. The range of normal hearing is from 0 dB to 25 dB. The further away from the range of normal hearing your test results fall, the greater your degree of hearing loss.

A distribution of the sounds of speech is shown on the audiogram in Figure 1-2. You can see that the vowels are low in frequency and the consonants are distributed over the low-, middle-, and high-frequency ranges. Often, people will be able to hear different pitched sounds at different loudness levels. This affects how the person will be able to hear speech. People who have a high-frequency loss will often complain that they know when someone is speaking to them, but that they cannot hear clearly what the words are. They will often complain of words sounding muffled, especially when they are listening in the presence of background noise.

A person with a high-frequency loss may also have difficulty hearing the sound of a telephone bell, a bird chirping, or a cricket, but have little difficulty hearing a male voice or someone speaking on the phone.

Understanding the implications of the type and degree of hearing loss you have can help you to cope better with the challenges it presents.

If the words being said at any moment contain a large number

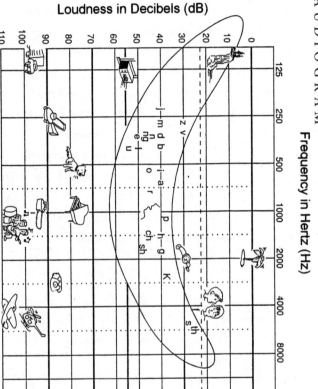

FIGURE 1-2

THE SPEECH AUDIOGRAM

of sounds that your hearing loss cuts out, you may have blanks to fill in so that you can figure out the message. If the topic changes and the words contain more of the sounds that are in your audible range, then you may be able to understand much more. This may make your hearing ability appear inconsistent, both to yourself and to others. Others may tell you, "You only hear what you want to hear."

Different types of hearing losses result in varying degrees of difficulty hearing the words that are being said. If your hearing ability is within normal range, it is expected that you would have no difficulty hearing the sounds in the speech spectrum shown in Figure 1-2. If, however, your marks fall below the range of normal hearing, you may see which of the speech sounds you are not able to hear.

9. How Does My Hearing Test Differ from the Tests of Others?

Each person's hearing ability is individual, just as each person is different. Some people hear better in the low frequencies; others hear better in the high frequencies, and others have a sharp sloping hearing loss. The results of each person's audiological evaluation (hearing test) are unique. A few sample audiometric configurations can be seen in Figures 1-3 through 1-9. Based on the explanations in Question 8, you can see how the individuals with these audiometric configurations would be affected differently. Some would be able to hear the consonants but not the vowels *(e.g., Figure 1-2)*. A person with a sharply sloping high frequency loss resulting from exposure to loud noise *(Figure 1-6)* would not be able to hear consonants and as a result would not be able to hear clearly in many communication situations.

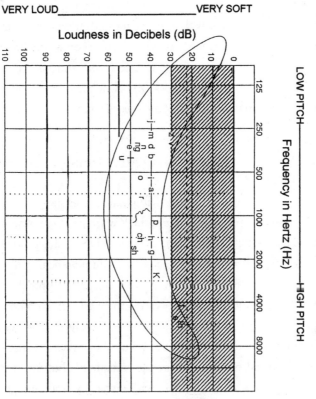

FIGURE 1-3

AN AUDIOGRAM SHOWING A MILD HEARING LOSS

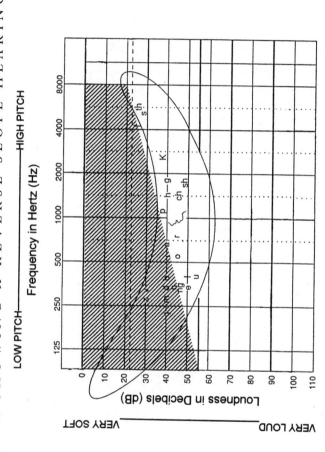

FIGURE 1-4
AN AUDIOGRAM SHOWING A REVERSE SLOPE HEARING LOSS

FIGURE 1-5

AN AUDIOGRAM SHOWING A MILD-MODERATE HEARING LOSS

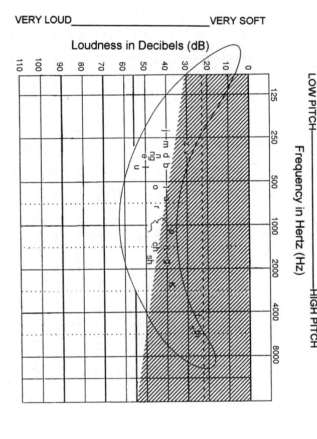

FIGURE 1-6
AN AUDIOGRAM SHOWING A NOISE-INDUCED HEARING LOSS

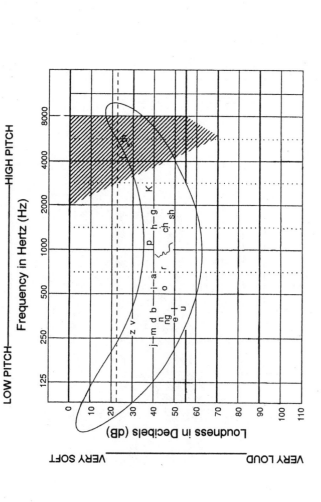

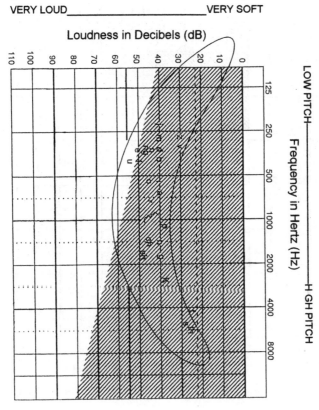

FIGURE 1-7 ....

AN AUDIOGRAM SHOWING MODERATE-SEVERE HEARING LOSS

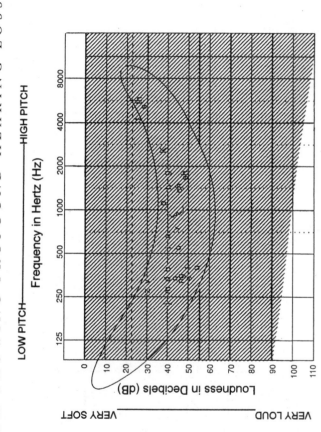

FIGURE 1-8
AN AUDIOGRAM SHOWING PROFOUND HEARING LOSS

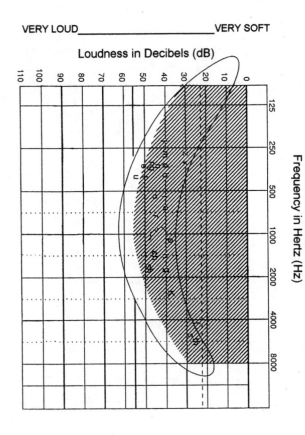

FIGURE 1-9 ......

AN AUDIOGRAM SHOWING A "COOKIE-BITE" HEARING LOSS

10. How Is Hearing Loss Described?

A hearing loss may be described in either words or numbers. Expressions such as "stone deaf" are incorrect because most people have some remaining hearing even if it's slight, and the expression "deaf and dumb" is misleading because deaf people do have the ability to communicate with sign language or with oral speech, although the inexperienced listener may find it difficult to understand them. People who are born with a severe hearing loss have difficulty learning to speak normally because they simply cannot hear other people's voices that well and therefore cannot imitate them, which is necessary in the process of developing speech. They are also unable to hear their own voices well when they try to speak. They often use sign language to facilitate communication.

The scientific method for measuring hearing loss (and sound in general) is in decibels (dB). Table 1-1 notes an approximate relationship between the decibel level of a hearing loss and the degree of difficulty it may cause.

TABLE 1-1 ·

THE EFFECT OF DIFFERENT DEGREES OF HEARING LOSS

Decibels of Hearing Loss	Degree of Impairment	Practical Effect on Hearing
0–25 dB	Normal	Little effect
26–40 dB	Mild	Difficulty with quiet voices
41–55 dB	Moderate	Difficulty with many voices
56–70 dB	Moderate-severe	Difficulty with most voices
71–90 dB	Severe	Cannot hear speech without a hearing aid
Over 91 dB	Profound	Can hear little even with a hearing aid

The varying degrees of hearing loss are drawn on the audiogram in Figure 1-1. The term *hard of hearing* is used if a person's degree of loss is in the mild to severe range, and the term *deaf* is used if the test results are in the profound range with little usable, residual hearing.

At times people may be told their hearing loss as a percentage, such as, "You have a 40 percent loss." This may seem easier to understand, but it is not a correct way to describe hearing since decibels cannot be converted in this way. One hundred decibels represents considerable hearing loss, but it definitely does not mean total deafness, and if this is the diagnosis it would certainly be advantageous to try out hearing aids for some hearing help.

For purposes of compensation for hearing lost in a noisy work environment, the percentage of "disability" can be calculated, but a 100 percent estimate of disability does not equal total deafness.

11. Are There Different Types of Hearing Loss?

There are two main types of hearing loss. *Conductive hearing loss* results in a loss of loudness. Someone with a conductive hearing loss is probably inclined to speak in a relatively quiet voice because when we speak, part of the sound of our own voice is transmitted directly through our head bone into our inner ear. Since we regulate the loudness of our voice by the way we hear ourselves, people with a conductive loss have a normal inner ear and hear their own voice louder than the voices of others. People with a conductive loss can generally hear and understand well in noisy surroundings because the conductive loss cushions them from the loud environmental sounds, and they benefit from the fact that everyone is speaking more loudly. Basically, for people with a conductive hearing loss sounds are just not loud enough to be heard well. This can be overcome by amplifying the sound and can often be remedied by medical or surgical techniques.

The second main type, *sensori-neural hearing loss,* leads not only to a loss of loudness but of clarity as well. This condition is sometimes incorrectly referred to as *nerve deafness,* and there is generally no medical or surgical help available for sensori-neural hearing loss. People with a sensori-neural hearing loss speak loudly, generally have more trouble understanding speech, and are especially bothered trying to understand speech in the presence of background noise. Often, people with sensori-neural hearing loss have an increased intolerance to loud sounds *(see Question 14)*.

One development that has occurred for profound sensori-neural hearing loss is the cochlear implant. *See Question 32, "Would an Operation Help?" and Question 67, "What Are Cochlear Implants?" for more information.*

Correcting the lack of clarity that may be associated with a sensori-neural hearing loss is not completely possible by amplifying sounds. It is important to be aware of this difference between a conductive and sensori-neural hearing loss. This helps you to understand why some people with hearing loss seem to manage so much better than others.

12. How Does the Ear Work?

The ear is divided into three parts: the outer, middle, and inner ear *(Figure 1-10)*.

The outer ear (3) includes the pinna (auricle) and the ear canal (4). The purpose of the pinna is to collect sound, which is then passed through the ear canal to the eardrum. Near its entrance, the surface of the ear canal is covered with small hairs and wax glands to protect the canal and to prevent dirt, insects, and anything else from entering. The ear canal is about one and a half inches long.

The middle ear is made up of the eardrum (5); the ossicles (the smallest bones in the body), which include the hammer (6), the anvil (7), and the stirrup (8); and the cavity that contains them. The function of the middle ear is to pass along to the inner ear the very small movements of the eardrum caused by the pressure of the sound waves.

The Eustachian tube (9) connects the middle ear cavity to the back of the throat and functions to equalize the air pressure in the middle ear.

FIGURE 1-10 ......

THE ANATOMY OF THE EAR

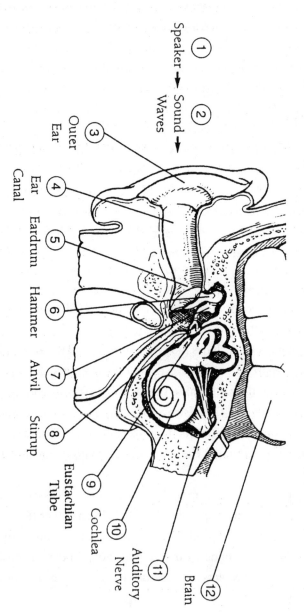

① Speaker → Sound Waves →

② Outer Ear

③ Ear Canal

④ Eardrum

⑤ Hammer

⑥ Anvil

⑦ Stirrup

⑧ Eustachian Tube

⑨ Cochlea

⑩ Auditory Nerve

⑪ Brain

⑫

The inner ear includes the cochlea (10), which is an extremely small, snail-shaped organ (about the size of a dried pea), which houses several thousand delicate hair cells. Here the vibrations received from the middle ear are changed into electrical signals that pass along the auditory nerve (11) to the brain (12), where the message is received and interpreted.

13. Do Many People Have Head Noises?

The condition of head noises, known as *tinnitus,* is quite common and experienced by an estimated 36 million Americans. Tinnitus can be pronounced two different ways: *"TIN-a-tus"* or *"Tin-EYE-tus."* Both pronunciations are correct. Tinnitus is a symptom, not a disease, and is frequently related to a disorder of the inner ear or auditory nerve. The noises may be heard in the head or in one ear or in both ears. Sometimes people with tinnitus have a hearing problem as well, but often their hearing is normal.

There are two types of tinnitus: subjective tinnitus, which is audible only to the person experiencing it; and objective tinnitus, which is actually audible to another person as well as to the person who is experiencing it. Nearly everyone experiences ringing in the ears at some time—particularly after exposure to loud noise, something we all should avoid.

In addition to loud noise exposure, the causes of tinnitus include:

- Alcohol and nicotine used to excess
- Aspirin taken in heavy doses
- Caffeine
- Earwax that is impacted or resting on the eardrum
- High blood pressure
- Hardening of the arteries

- Infection or inflammation in the ear canal or middle ear

- Certain medications

- Meniere's disease

- Meningitis

- Otosclerosis

- A tumor on the auditory nerve

There is no cure for tinnitus at the present time. In fact, it is not usually possible to say exactly where in the hearing system it is produced. Some people adapt to the noises and learn to ignore them, while others find them almost unbearable. They are often worse at night when you are tired, before you go to sleep, and first thing in the morning. It is important not to be alarmed; the noises are usually not a sign of a serious medical condition. However, it is advisable that you have a thorough medical checkup to determine if there is any treatable medical problem causing your tinnitus.

A small number of clinics specialize in the treatment of tinnitus. Check with your physician or contact the American Tinnitus Association *(see Question 107, "What Other Organizations Provide Help?")* for a list of such facilities in your area. Treatment may include:

- Hearing aids

- A masker, a small device that looks like a hearing aid and generates gentle rushing sounds that may cover up or mask the much less pleasant sound in the head

- An adjustment of diet

- Habituation therapy

- Cognitive therapy

- Relaxation training

■ Biofeedback

Self-help groups, run by people who share this problem, are being formed in many parts of the country as well. Check with the American Tinnitus Association and SHHH (Self Help for Hard of Hearing People, Inc.). *See Chapter 6 for more information.*

14. How Can I Be Hard of Hearing and Yet Be Painfully Sensitive to Noise?

Although it does seem odd, many people with hearing loss are unusually touchy about noise. This is one of the characteristics of a sensori-neural loss and is called *recruitment*. It means that there is an abnormally rapid buildup of the sensation of the loudness of a sound. Therefore, as soon as a sound becomes loud enough to be heard, a slight increase in loudness might bring pain. This explains why certain levels of loudness hurt some people's ears, even though other people are perfectly comfortable with the same sounds.

It is very important that a person's tolerance level to loud sounds is measured when hearing aids are fit. Then, hearing aids can be adjusted to keep all sounds below the threshold for pain. New technology in hearing aid design can control for this problem and can increase people's satisfaction and comfort with their hearing aids.

15. How Are Dizziness and Hearing Loss Related?

The cochlea in the inner ear connects with the semicircular canals, which help to provide our sense of balance. There is a condition that results in hearing loss, tinnitus, and dizziness: Meniere's disease (named after a famous French physician). This condition can be very distressing and requires medical treatment. Attacks of dizziness may occur at unpredictable intervals, and the hearing loss and tinnitus may fluctuate. Sometimes hearing will return to normal even without any treatment.

Attacks of dizziness or loss of balance should be taken

seriously and you should always obtain medical advice. There are many conditions that can lead to dizziness, some of which are connected with hearing. Therefore, if you suffer from this problem, your family physician may refer you to an otologist or otolaryngologist (an ear specialist).

16. Can Hearing Loss Affect the Voice and the Way People Speak?

This will usually happen only if your hearing loss becomes severe. Most people with a relatively minor loss can be reassured that their voice and manner of speech will remain quite normal. One problem may be that you may not be able to tell if you are talking too loudly or too softly. Hearing aids should eliminate this problem. Another problem may result if you have lost hearing in a specific frequency range, making it difficult for you to hear how you are pronouncing certain speech sounds. When we speak, we use vowels and consonants. The vowels are lower in frequency (pitch) and are heard in the lower frequency range *(indicated on Figure 1-2)*. Consonants are heard in the higher frequencies. If you are not able to clearly hear some sounds, you may not be able to pronounce them clearly.

Hearing is the main channel through which we develop language skills. If a child is born with a severe hearing loss or becomes severely hearing impaired before learning to speak, it is likely that the quality of the child's voice and clarity of speech will be affected. The child will have to be taught words and the principles of language. Such children may be referred to as *prelingually deaf,* while people who lose their hearing after they have acquired speech are referred to as *postlingually deafened.*

17. How Can I Explain My Hearing Loss to Others?

Become familiar with the information in this chapter about how to read an audiogram and then plot the results of your last hearing test on the blank audiogram in Figure 1-11. This will help you to understand your degree of hearing loss as well as just what sounds you have difficulty hearing. Explaining this to others with whom you communicate will help them to understand why you hear some sounds and miss others.

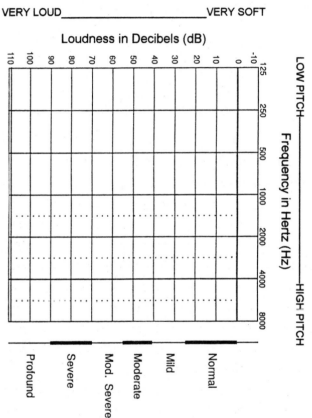

FIGURE 1-11

A BLANK AUDIOGRAM

CHAPTER TWO

The *Causes* of *Hearing Loss*

18. What Can Cause Hearing Loss?

The simplest cause of hearing loss is a buildup of wax in the ear canal. If this wax, called *cerumen,* completely blocks the ear canal, you might experience a very noticeable loss of hearing. Wax is produced naturally in the outer ear canal and some people produce much more wax than others. People who wear hearing aids may have an increase in the amount of wax in the ear canals since the hearing aid or earmold tends to reduce the amount of natural ventilation to the ear. Fortunately, in most cases the wax is easily removed by a physician (either with a probe or by flushing with water).

Other items pushed too far into the ear canal, such as cotton, can create the same effect. Even though some people use cotton or other items in an attempt to clean the ear canal, the adage that says that "you shouldn't put anything smaller than your elbow into your ear" should be followed. Using hairpins, matchsticks, or cotton swabs can cause the wax to be pushed deeper into the canal beyond the point where it will naturally leave *(see Question 33).*

A cold or a sinus infection may cause you to experience some hearing loss *(see Question 26)*. These create a slight fullness that should disappear when you get over the cold or infection. If you fly or travel in the mountains, you may also experience a minor degree of hearing loss due to the difference in pressure between the air in the middle ear and the outside air. This problem usually will disappear if you blow your nose, swallow, or chew gum.

Exposure to loud noise, even for a short period, can cause you to feel that your hearing ability is lessened, and you may also experience some tinnitus (ringing in the ears). Called a *temporary threshold shift*, this problem usually goes away after a period of time once you are out of the noisy environment. Too much exposure to loud noise can lead in time to a permanent hearing loss *(see Question 23)*.

As we live longer, the chances that we will experience some reduction in our ability to hear is high. It is estimated that on average one in ten people have some degree of hearing loss. Over the age of sixty, the estimate changes to one in four, and over the age of seventy, it's one in two.

A common cause of conductive hearing loss (affecting the middle ear) is otosclerosis, a condition in which one of the small bones in the middle ear (the stapes in the ossicular chain) is affected with a bony growth. An operation called a *stapedectomy* may be performed to overcome this problem.

Infection in the middle ear can cause a buildup of fluid in the middle ear cavity, leading to a temporary hearing loss and possibly a discharge from the ear. Perforations of the eardrum (tympanic membrane) can also lead to conductive hearing loss.

Conductive hearing loss is usually medically or surgically correctable, but sensori-neural hearing loss is usually irreversible. Sensori-neural hearing loss can be caused by a wide range of viral infections, such as measles, mumps, or meningitis. Certain medications can also cause an irreversible hearing loss *(see Question 24)*, as can exposure to loud noise or a blow to the head.

19. Why Are Some Babies Born with Hearing Loss?

Various infectious diseases experienced by a woman when pregnant may result in one or more disabilities for the child . If a woman contracts the infectious disease rubella (German measles) during the first three months of pregnancy, there is a risk that the baby might be born with hearing loss. It is therefore strongly recommended that children be immunized early against the disease.

A difficult birth that results in the baby's receiving insufficient oxygen may cause hearing impairment. Because hearing loss can pass from one generation to the next, hereditary and genetic factors are also very important. Genetic counseling by a specialist who has knowledge about hearing loss is very important if you suspect a hereditary or genetic factor.

20. Do Earaches Matter?

Earaches do matter; they are an indication that something is wrong. They can be caused by such things as middle ear infections or the additional pressure of jaw pain. It is important to see a physician if an earache persists.

21. My Child Gets Ear Infections—What Can I Do?

An infection of the middle ear caused by bacteria is called *otitis media*. Otitis media is one of the most common causes of earache in young children. It is estimated that more than 60 percent of all children will have at least one episode of otitis media by age one; 80 percent will have an episode by age three; and one-third of all children will have three or more episodes. Your child may be feverish and irritable and may experience discomfort and pain. A runny nose or nasal congestion may occur along with temporary hearing loss. For many children, recurring infections are common and unavoidable because of their physiology. It is important that you follow your physician's instructions. The infection may be cured within approximately seven to ten days. For some children, if infections are frequent, your physician may recommend tubes.

22. Could Damage to the Eardrum Be Serious?

It is often thought that if the eardrum is damaged you will become totally deaf. This is not true. Damage to the eardrum in the form of a perforation or rupture will cause some hearing loss of the conductive type. If the eardrum does not heal naturally, an operation called *tympanoplasty* can bring about a repair. Ear, nose, and throat surgeons will sometimes deliberately make a small perforation in the eardrums of children or individuals who have a buildup of fluid in the middle ear. Called a *myringotomy*, this operation prevents the eardrum from closing since a small tube is inserted into the hole in the eardrum to provide ventilation of the middle ear and a path through which the thick fluid, often called *glue*, will escape.

If you have a perforation of the eardrum, you will need to use earplugs if you want to swim or bathe so that water does not enter the middle ear. These earplugs can be purchased at a drugstore or specially designed earplugs can be made from exact ear impressions by your audiologist or ear physician.

23. Can Noise Damage Hearing?

Excessive noise can cause hearing loss. Some people who have worked in noisy factories or served in the armed forces in combat have experienced a change in hearing ability. Legislation has been introduced to regulate the limits of the sound levels to protect people's hearing. The current limit is eighty-five decibels, about the level of a subway train. If the noise exceeds the limit, employers must provide ear protection in the form of plugs or muffs; cotton is not effective. It is very important to follow the instructions of the health safety officer or nurse in your place of work. If there are areas that have been measured to be loud enough to cause damage to your hearing, wear ear protection.

It is also necessary to consider the amount of time spent in the noisy environment. The louder the noise, the shorter the time you should be exposed to it. Unfortunately, some people are more susceptible than others to this type of hearing loss, and there is no way to predict their susceptibility until it is too late. If your work or hobbies put you at risk, it is a good idea to be tested regularly to monitor and prevent any problems.

Many sounds can damage hearing. For example, if you fire a gun or a rifle or use a chainsaw, a lawnmower or a snow blower, you need to wear ear protection. If you attend rock concerts or play in a band or an orchestra, remember that exposure to loud sounds can damage hearing and it doesn't matter if it's the Beatles, Beethoven, or the blues. Ear protection should be worn in any situation where noise levels exceed 85 dB. A good way to determine if it is too loud is to see if you have difficulty hearing someone speaking next to you while the music is playing. If so, use ear protectors (foam earplugs available over the counter at the drugstore), or at least limit the amount of time you are exposed to the loud music by taking periodic breaks to give your ears a rest. There are special custom-made ear protectors that are designed in such a way that musicians still can hear the sounds of music but at a reduced level. Check with your audiologist to arrange to have impressions taken.

It is also important to use personal radios and stereo cassette or CD players with earphones carefully. If they are too loud, they can damage your hearing permanently. It is best not to set the volume beyond the halfway point; if a passerby can hear the sound of the music, it is too loud. It is important to remember that such damage to the hearing mechanism is cumulative. You may not be aware of it, but over time with frequent exposure to loud sounds, the loss is added to whatever loss you acquire as you get older.

Warning signs of exposure to sound levels that may be dangerous to your hearing include:

- You have ringing or buzzing in your ears after exposure to noise.

- You have pain in your ears after exposure to noise.

- You notice that sounds seem muffled.

- You have difficulty hearing quiet sounds after a period of exposure to loud sounds.

- You feel a fullness in your ears.

It is important to protect your hearing. You can do this by moving away from the sound source and, when possible, turning down the volume. There are also noise cancellation devices available that reduce the low-pitched sounds in the environment (such as the sounds you hear when riding on a plane). These reduce fatigue and allow you to hear speech more clearly. Whenever possible, take rest periods to reduce the cumulative effect of loud noise. Avoid leisure activities with high noise exposure and wear ear protection devices. Remember, you can prevent hearing loss by protecting your ears.

24. Can Medications Damage Hearing?

There are a number of drugs that are *ototoxic,* which means that they are capable of damaging the hearing system. Some of these are powerful life-saving medications, but others are widely used remedies. Even aspirin, if taken in large quantities, can affect your hearing. Some medications can cause tinnitus, so if you are taking medication that seems to be causing a dullness in your hearing or noises in your head, tell your doctor. Some drugs will cause a temporary loss, but with others the loss could be permanent.

25. Can Accidents Damage Hearing?

Accidents that involve head injuries may cause hearing loss due to damage to the nerves that carry signals to the brain or damage to the part of the brain that receives the auditory signals, called the *auditory cortex.* A blast may rupture the eardrum, and large changes in pressure experienced by divers may cause risk of hearing loss. A severe blow to the head might result in some reduction in hearing ability.

26. Why Is My Hearing Affected when I Have a Cold?

A simple cold can often affect hearing, usually by causing a swelling of the Eustachian tube. This may result in pressure in the middle ear or even an accumulation of fluid in the middle ear. These changes may fluctuate a good deal and may be relieved by decongestants. When the cold goes away, the hearing loss almost always disappears.

27. Why Is Hearing Loss Confined to One Ear in Some People?

A loss of hearing in one ear is called a *unilateral hearing loss*. It might be the result of a blow to the head, a tumor, ear infections, or disease. Some "childhood" diseases, such as mumps or measles, may cause a high fever that results in damage to the hearing in one ear. A unilateral hearing loss makes it harder to locate the directions that sound is coming from. This can make it more dangerous for you when you are in traffic. It can also make it harder for you to understand speech in a group conversation or when there is background noise. How you position yourself while driving or at social gatherings can help you to follow conversations. You should also try a hearing aid to help improve hearing performance. Either a standard unit or one called a CROS (Contralateral Routing of Signals) instrument might be helpful. The CROS hearing aid allows speech to be understood from the affected ear by placing a microphone-type receiver over that ear; the receiver then transmits the sounds to the better ear This can help you to hear conversation when there is background noise, and after a period of time some users develop a sense of sound directionality.

28. Why Do We Lose Our Hearing as We Get Older?

As we live longer and grow older, our bodies tend to slow down. Our hearing and our sight might function less efficiently. Hearing loss that occurs as we get older has a medical name: *presbyacusis*. This is a sensori-neural loss and is primarily due to changes in the inner ear and to some extent in the nerve that leads to the brain. The loss of hearing is usually gradual and it affects most people, some more than others. Being unable to hear high-pitched sounds is what most people notice first. This makes it harder to understand certain words, especially when they are spoken by a woman with a high-pitched voice or by young children. Often, the person with this type of hearing loss is not aware of this connection and may blame others for mumbling or not speaking clearly. It is often only when others point out such misunderstandings that the person realizes it would be a good idea to get a hearing check up. It is important not to wait until the occasional difficulties with understanding conversations become real communication problems. Unfortunately, too many people put up with hearing that is becoming worse before they seek help. So much can be done to assist those who have difficulty hearing. It is wise to check the options available.

CHAPTER THREE

The *Treatment* of *Hearing Loss*

29. How Is Treatment Available?

Under normal circumstances if you experience a loss of hearing, you should first visit your family physician, who will examine you and if necessary refer you to a specialist for further evaluation and care. If you have had no history of ear infections or medical problems with your ears, your family physician will recommend that you have your hearing checked by an audiologist. If necessary, the audiologist will provide you with information about means of hearing assistance, which include hearing aids, assistive listening devices and systems, and aural rehabilitative care.

If you ever experience a sudden, severe loss of hearing, you should see your ear, nose, and throat physician (otolaryngologist) as soon as possible. If you do not have an otolaryngologist, go to the emergency room of the nearest hospital. Swift treatment may restore your hearing.

30. Is Treatment for Hearing Loss Any Better than It Was Twenty Years Ago?

The answer to this question is a definite yes. So much can be done medically, surgically, or with hearing aids and other assistive devices that can reduce the problems of hearing loss. Newborn infants can be evaluated if hearing loss is suspected, and efforts to correct the problem can be done swiftly so that needless delays do not interfere with speech, language and learning.

Medications are available that can correct or control infection. Surgery can reconstruct parts of the ear to improve hearing. An electrode can be implanted into the cochlea in the inner ear of persons who have lost almost all of their hearing ability; this artificially allows them to hear again. Research is being done to unravel the mystery of the inner ear hair cell regeneration and its potential application to humans as a means of treating deafness.

31. Can Medication Be Helpful?

Medications are used to provide treatment for many problems related to the ear and hearing. They are used to treat infections or an underlying condition. Usually, medications are not prescribed on a long-term basis; once the problem is cleared up, the medication is stopped. There are no medications that will cure a sensori-neural hearing loss ("nerve deafness").

32. Would an Operation Help?

Currently, most operations for hearing loss are done to correct problems in the middle ear. Your otolaryngologist can determine if an operation would help to correct your hearing loss. One common condition is called *otosclerosis*. This is a result of a bony growth forming at the base of the stapes, preventing the movement of the ossicles in the middle ear. An operation called a *stapedectomy* replaces the stapes with a metal or plastic piston and has a good rate of success in restoring hearing to near normal levels.

Before the days when antibiotics were available, the *mastoid operation* was quite common to treat infections of the middle ear that could lead to an abscess forming in the mastoid bone. Fortunately, today mastoid operations are relatively rare.

If the eardrum has a perforation, an operation called a *tympanoplasty* can be done to close the hole. Hearing can be restored almost to normal when this operation is successful.

FIGURE 3-1

THE COCHLEAR IMPLANT

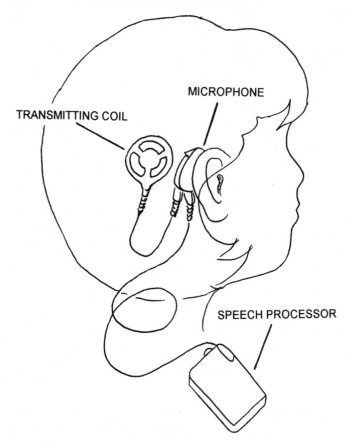

MICROPHONE

TRANSMITTING COIL

SPEECH PROCESSOR

The cochlear implant *(above)* is an operation that provides some hearing to a person who has a profound sensori-neural hearing loss. This operation is useful for people who receive little or no assistance from hearing aids. An electrode is implanted into the cochlea and, with the help of a signal processing unit worn externally, the user gains an awareness of sounds that otherwise could not be heard. Some cochlear implant recipients do experience significant improvement in understanding speech as well *(see Question 67)*.

This summary includes the most common operations, but there are a wide range of other operations for specialized cases. It is important to check with your physician to see if you require any operation to improve your hearing.

33. What Can Be Done for Earwax?

The skin of the outer part of the ear canal has special glands that produce earwax. This is supposed to prevent dust, sand, and insects from reaching the eardrum. Usually, the wax accumulates a bit, dries up, and falls out of the ear, carrying the dust with it. When earwax has accumulated so much that it blocks the ear and maybe even your hearing, you may need to have it removed by your physician or audiologist. There are products available from your pharmacy that you may obtain to clean out your ears yourself. Do not attempt this if you know your ear is infected or if you have a hole in your eardrum. Follow the directions carefully and be certain to place one eyedropper of rubbing alcohol into the ear canal afterward. The alcohol absorbs the water, dries out quickly, and destroys any bacteria or fungus that might be present.

34. Can Hearing Aids Help?

For those people who cannot benefit from medical or surgical treatment for hearing loss, hearing aids can provide practical help. This is especially true for most sensori-neural hearing losses, contrary to the myth that nerve losses cannot be helped with hearing aids. Hearing aids can provide a good deal of assistance in helping you to improve your ability to hear. While they do not restore perfect hearing, they can help you to hear better; that's why they're called *aids*. They can make communication easier, and because of this they can make life more comfortable and pleasant. You should not put off getting help if you are having difficulty hearing. Modern hearing aids take advantage of the newest technology and can make a big difference in your life.

35. Can Assistive Listening Devices and Systems Help Me if I Live Alone and Am Hard of Hearing?

Assistive listening devices and systems (ALDS) can help. An ALDS is defined as any device other than a standard hearing aid that is designed to improve a hearing-impaired person's ability to communicate and to function more independently either by transmitting amplified sound more directly from its source to the listener or by transforming it into a tactile or visual signal. Many of these devices, such as alarm clocks connected to bed vibrators or to flashing lights, telephone alarms, and doorbell alarms, have been available for many years. Other items, such as television listening systems, personal one-on-one amplifiers, FM transmission systems, telecommunication devices, and wearable tactile alarms have more recently entered the marketplace. *See Chapter 5 for detailed information about ALDS.*

36. What Else Can Be Done?

Besides medical care, hearing aids, and assistive listening devices and systems, a great deal can be done to alleviate the communication problems associated with a hearing loss. Classes called *aural rehabilitation* include training and orientation in the adjustment and use of hearing aids, exercises in various communication strategies, and speechreading (lipreading) practice. These are described in Chapter 6.

37. What Does the Future Hold for People with Hearing Impairment?

Research is being done on hair cell regeneration in chickens and other animals, which scientists hope one day will lead the way to repairing the damaged hair cells in the inner ear of humans. Technology offers the possibility of voice recognition systems that promise to ease communication for people with limited hearing ability. In addition, other assistive devices are being developed to facilitate greater independence and improved communication.

CHAPTER FOUR

Hearing Aids

38. Do I Need Hearing Aids?

Do you have trouble hearing the telephone or doorbell ring? Does your family say that you play the television too loudly? Do you sometimes fail to understand words clearly? Do you find that other people seem to mumble? If you answer yes to any of these questions, you may benefit from the help of hearing aids. Hearing aids are miniature amplifiers that do not affect your hearing loss, but do make it easier for you to hear. Often, others may notice that you are having difficulty hearing before you are aware of it. It is a good idea to get hearing help sooner rather than later if you find yourself struggling to hear since you do not want to cut yourself off from others.

You may wish to take The Five-Minute Hearing Test. You will find it in Appendix 7.

39. Would a Hearing Aid Help if I Have a "Nerve Loss"?

Yes, a hearing aid can provide you with some hearing help even if you have what is called a "nerve loss." It is an often repeated myth that people who have "nerve deafness" cannot be helped with hearing aids. Nothing is further from the truth. The majority of people who do use hearing aids today have a sensori-neural hearing loss (popularly labeled "nerve deafness"), since medical and surgical techniques can usually correct a conductive hearing loss *(see Question 11)*. If you have been told in the past that you cannot benefit from hearing aids because of "nerve deafness," check again.

40. What Hearing Aids Are Available?

There are more than thirty manufacturers of hearing aids in the world today. Since they each build several models, the result is a large number of products on the market from which to choose. However, all of these products can be placed into four categories depending upon where they are worn. These are:

1. The body aid

2. The eyeglass unit

3. The behind-the-ear model

4. The in-the-ear type

Although their appearance may vary, all hearing aids have a similar set of functional parts: a microphone, an amplifier with volume control, and a receiver. The microphone converts sound waves into electrical energy. The amplifier increases the strength of the electrical signal, boosting the energy. The receiver converts or changes the amplified electrical signal back into sound energy. Acoustic features of the instruments can be programmed using microchip technology. A battery provides the power source to the hearing aid. The size of the battery depends on the style and size of the hearing aid. *(Figure 4-1)*

FIGURE 4-1

COMPONENTS OF A HEARING AID WITH BATTERIES

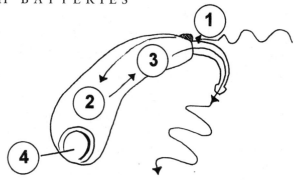

1. MICROPHONE —sound waves enter and are converted into electrical energy

2. AMPLIFIER —increases the strength of the electrical signal, boosting energy

3. RECEIVER —changes the electrical signal back into amplified sound waves

4. POWER SOURCE —the battery is the hearing aid's power source

HEARING AID BATTERIES

AA   675   13   312   230 or 10

One style may be more suitable for one person's type of hearing loss than another. In addition to shape and style, there are internal differences between hearing aids, such as in the range of tones that are amplified, the loudness of the sounds that can be delivered to the ear, and the way the amplification system processes the sound. Digital technology is being used in hearing instruments today. Hearing aids can be set specifically to meet your special hearing needs.

Fewer than 2 percent of the hearing aids fitted today are body-worn aids since technology has miniaturized circuitry to put a similar amount of power once only available in the body aid into a behind-the-ear instrument (and even in some of the in-the-ear hearing aids). The body-worn aid includes a small box (smaller than a cigarette pack), which holds the amplifier and microphone to which is attached a cord with a button receiver *(Figure 4-2)*. A specially molded earpiece is then snapped to the receiver.

FIGURE 4-2 ·······

A BODY HEARING AID

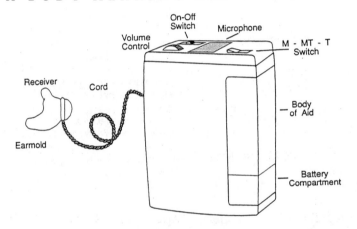

An eyeglass hearing aid has the microphone, amplifier, and receiver built into the temple piece of the eyeglasses. Attached to the temple piece is a plastic tube with an earmold that is worn in the ear *(Figure 4-3)*. Though still manufactured, this model is not very popular since combining both types of equipment (for vision and hearing) can be complicated and might not be practical. For example, if one broke, you'd be without the other.

FIGURE 4-3 ··

AN EYEGLASS HEARING AID

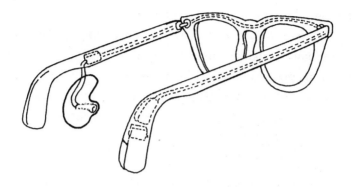

The behind-the-ear hearing aid is worn over the ear with a plastic tube attached to an earmold placed in the ear *(Figure 4-4)*. About 20 percent of the hearing aids fitted today in the United States are behind-the-ear instruments. This style hearing aid can be set so as to provide help to persons with a very mild to profound loss of hearing.

FIGURE 4-4 ··

A BEHIND-THE-EAR HEARING AID

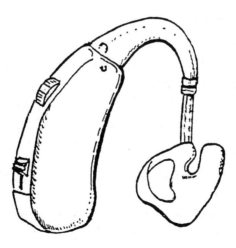

The in-the-ear hearing aid can be built in a variety of sizes depending upon the amount of power you need as well as your dexterity and how much you wish to pay. The original in-the-ear hearing aid fills the entire concha portion of the ear *(see Figure 1-10 in Chapter 1)*. It has been around longer than the other in-the-ear models, and since it is the largest, it is made of the heaviest weight plastic and is usually more durable.

A variety of styles of in-the-ear instruments include the low profile, half-shell, in-the-canal, mini-canal, and completely-in-the-canal hearing aids *(see Figure 4-5)*. There are advantages and disadvantages to each. They vary in the amount of power and durability as well as in the size of the controls. It is important to discuss the pros and cons of each style as well as the technology with your audiologist. Keep in mind that the most suitable hearing aid is not necessarily the most powerful, the least visible, or the one recommended by your friend. Also, remember that just because a hearing aid costs more, it is not necessarily going to work better for you.

Each in-the-ear instrument is built to your specific amplification needs based on the results of your hearing tests. An impression of your ear is taken so that the custom-built units will fit you comfortably.

41. What Is an Earmold?

An earmold is an important part of a complete hearing aid system connecting the hearing aid to the ear. It is necessary if you wear a body aid, an eyeglass instrument, or a behind-the-ear hearing aid *(see Figures 4-2, 4-3, and 4-4)*. Earmolds are usually custom-molded to insure a good fit. They are prepared from an impression taken of each ear, similar to the way dentures are made.

Earmolds come in a variety of styles and materials depending on your type and degree of hearing loss. The choice can affect the amount and quality of sound channeled from the hearing aid into

FIGURE 4-5 ·

IN-THE-EAR, IN-THE-CANAL, AND COMPLETELY IN-THE-CANAL HEARING AIDS

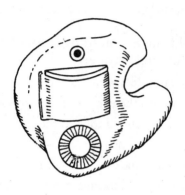

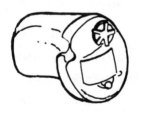

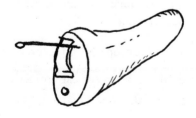

your ear. The choice is generally made by your dispenser based on your needs.

Your ear will change shape as you grow taller or vary your weight. Children's earmolds need to be checked by the dispenser on a regular basis to guarantee a proper fit. If your weight has changed, be certain to have the fit of your earmolds checked as well.

42. How Should the Earmold or In-the-Ear Hearing Aid Be Inserted Properly?

Make certain the earmold/hearing aid is clean and free of earwax before inserting it into the ear. Hold the earmold/hearing aid upright with the nib pointed toward the ear canal. Using the thumb and index finger, pinch the earmold/hearing aid securely. Insert the nib snug into the ear canal. Turn the earmold/hearing aid back and then forward, locking it into place. Press to ensure that it is seated into place. If you have a behind-the-ear instrument, lift upward and place it behind your ear. Now, turn on the hearing aid, setting the volume, if necessary, to a comfortable listening level.

43. Can I Use My Earmolds as Noise Protectors?

Even the most tight-fitting earmolds do not provide as much protection in loud noise as do commercial ear protectors. Always protect your ears from excessive noise insult by using quality, well-fitting, specifically designed ear protection.

44. Why Do Some Hearing Aids Squeal?

A high-pitched squeal will come from the hearing aid for one or a combination of these reasons:

1. You have not inserted it properly and securely into your ear.

2. The hearing aid does not fit your ear correctly (if you have gained size or weight or if the plastic material has shrunk).

3. The tubing on your earmold has hardened or cracked.

4. The volume of the hearing aid is too high.

5. The hearing aid is malfunctioning.

This whistle is often not heard by the person wearing the hearing aid, but it may be annoying to others. When this whistle occurs, it reduces the effectiveness of the hearing aid. The problem can be corrected, so see your hearing aid dispenser. Remember, a hearing aid is not supposed to squeal when it is in your ear.

45. Are Hearing Aids Uncomfortable and Might They Be Irritating?

When you first get your hearing aids, you will certainly know that you have them in your ears. You will be aware of the piece of plastic and you may even feel their weight. However, after a short adjustment time, you will not be aware of the hearing aids in your ears. They are not supposed to hurt. If the hearing aid or earmold is uncomfortable after you have worn it for a week or two, contact your hearing aid dispenser for assistance. They are available to provide you with this continued service.

For a long time before you actually noticed that you were having some difficulty understanding speech, you had already lost some of the ability to hear such sounds as the hum of a fluorescent light, the rustling of paper, the drip of a faucet, the click of your footsteps, or the squeak of a chair. You had grown accustomed to living in a quieter world, not hearing loud sounds such as a horn honking, a dog barking, or the sound of your car engine. Your new hearing aids are amplifiers that make all sounds in the environment louder, not just the ones you'd want to hear. At first, you may find the noises irritating. It is similar to suddenly having a strong light shone into your eyes when you've gotten used to the dark. Following a gradual adjustment schedule can reduce some of this auditory shock and help you to slowly become comfortable with your new world of sound.

46. Are Hearing Aids Adjustable?

Hearing aids can be adjusted internally by your hearing aid dispenser to control the amount and type of amplification to give you the amount and quality of sound that will benefit you the most. Some hearing aids have a user-operated volume (or gain) control. Some volume controls are independent, as on the behind-the-ear hearing aid shown in Figure 4-4; others are integrated into the on-off switch, as shown on the in-the-ear model in Figure 4-5. Hearing aids can also be built for use with a hand-held remote control device to manipulate volume as well as other amplification qualities. For some individuals who cannot manage a variable volume control, a screw-set control can be built in and set by the dispenser.

Body-worn hearing aids usually have a tone control that can be adjusted by the user. The control may have the following markings:

1. "L" for the emphasis of low tones

2. "N" for the normal response

3. "H" for the emphasis of high tones as well as for reducing the effects of background noise when trying to listen to conversation

Some behind-the-ear hearing aids may have an "NS" control that is similar to the "H" control on the body-worn aid; it provides some reduction of background noise for the user in a conversational setting.

As hearing aids get smaller, fewer user-operated tone controls can be installed. New technology has delivered hearing instruments that, when programmed, require no further volume adjustment by the user or may be adjusted with a remote control. Called *programmable* or *digital* hearing aids or hearing systems, these units integrate microchip circuitry into the hearing aid, providing the user with ease of use and a more comfortable sound quality in varying listening environments.

47. Do All Hearing Aids Need Batteries? How Long Do the Batteries Last?

Every hearing aid needs some form of electrical power except for the antique ear trumpet. Rechargeable batteries are sometimes used, and even solar cells are possible, but the majority of batteries used are disposable. Some disposable batteries can be recycled. Check with your dispenser about how you can do this.

Each manufacturer of hearing aid batteries uses a different letter code after the number of the battery displayed on the battery pack. For some, this will indicate if the battery is made of mercury or zinc. Generally, the zinc air-activated batteries will last longer than the mercury batteries. The important thing for you to remember when purchasing batteries is the number of the battery that fits your hearing aid.

Hearing aid battery life varies with the type of battery you use, the size of the battery needed for your hearing aid, the amount of power you need, and how much you wear your hearing aid. On average, the 675 zinc air-activated hearing aid battery will last about three weeks with a standard-type linear amplifier if you have a moderate loss of hearing and are using your hearing aid all day, every day. When using the programmable hearing instruments, expect a shorter use time per battery. Mercury batteries have an even shorter life expectancy. Generally, the size of the battery also affects the power capacity. *(The variety of battery sizes available are shown in Figure 4-1.)* Check with your dispenser to determine the most efficient battery for your use.

It is important to keep hearing aid batteries clearly marked and away from small children. Some children have mistaken hearing aid batteries for candy; some adults have mistaken them for medications. Hearing aid batteries can be poisonous if swallowed. See a doctor or call the National Button Battery Hotline collect at (202) 625-3333 if a hearing aid battery is swallowed. (You may want to post this number near your phone.) Tamper-free battery doors can be installed onto hearing aids to be used by small children to prevent this problem from occurring.

48. Will My Hearing Get Worse if I Use Hearing Aids?

Some people think that if you begin to use hearing aids you will become dependent on them and that your hearing will become worse. Hearing aids that are correctly fitted will not cause your hearing to deteriorate, but they will not prevent your hearing loss from becoming worse, either. For most people, changes in their hearing occur very slowly. In our noisy industrial society, nearly everybody realizes some reduction in hearing acuity as they grow older.

If your hearing aids are fit properly and you have adapted to using them on a full-time basis, you are getting optimum benefit from the instruments and you are wisely not switching from one level of hearing to another.

49. Are Two Instruments Better than One?

It is generally felt that if two hearing aids can be fit successfully, they should be used for optimum benefit. A binaural fitting (wearing hearing aids in both ears) makes it easier for the user to hear in noisy places such as in the car or in restaurants or at parties. When two hearing aids are worn, it is also easier for the user to tell from which direction sounds are coming. This help in localizing sound is very important for safety in traffic and in the environment in general and should not be overlooked. Sounds will be fuller and richer and have more depth for you if two hearing aids are properly fit and worn.

Some might feel that adapting to two hearing aids is twice as difficult as to one. With a slow, gradual wearing schedule and daily practice, it is possible for all hearing aid users to become adept at wearing their hearing aids and getting the most out of them. It is wise to keep in mind that it takes time to become skillful at wearing hearing aids. Most people need to progress gradually in adapting to regular, full-time hearing aid use.

50. How Do I Get Hearing Aids?

If you feel that you may need help with your hearing, begin by following the steps listed in Question 6. An audiological evaluation will provide information about the health of your ears and hearing system. Your audiologist will review your test results with you, specifying the type and degree of hearing loss you have as well as how the results affect your ability to communicate.

Depending on these results and on your particular communication and lifestyle needs, the audiologist will either suggest that you try hearing aids or that you wait until your need for hearing assistance increases. Most audiologists also dispense hearing aids, but if they do not they will recommend where you can obtain a thirty-day hearing aid trial before making a purchase. When you choose where you will purchase your hearing aids, consider the expertise and reputation of the dispenser as well as the dispenser's availability for follow-up care.

51. What Do I Do After I Get Hearing Aids?

It is important to realize that getting hearing aids is only a beginning step in learning to hear again. It takes time to get accustomed to having something in your ears and to adjust to the quality of sound provided by hearing instruments; for some, it takes a few months. If you have been losing your hearing over a period of time, you may have forgotten just how loud many sounds in our environment actually can be. You may find it useful to follow a gradual adjustment schedule as you adapt to wearing your hearing aids. You do not want to overtire yourself.

Generally, it is recommended that you begin wearing your hearing aids for short periods of time, for about a two-hour stretch three times each day in a quiet, nonstressful environment. Gradually increase your wearing time by about one hour each day in different environments so that after a period of two weeks you will be comfortable wearing your hearing aids all day, every day, from the time you awaken until you go to bed. Spend time getting acquainted with adjusting the controls on the hearing aids (if applicable) and practicing proper insertion for maximum comfort. Then, during your first experiences with the new amplified sounds, listen and identify what it is you think you are hearing, adjusting the volume to a level that is pleasing and not too loud. Notice what the different sounds are, identify them, and then file them in your memory to leave your attention free to listen to those sounds most important to you.

Vary your listening experiences from quiet to more challenging. After the first week of wearing your hearing aids in the quiet of your home, wear them when you are driving or going shopping. Begin to wear them in your work environment if it is not too noisy. By the third week, you should be ready to use the instruments in most life situations except, perhaps, at a party or at a very noisy restaurant. Give yourself time to gradually adapt to the very loud sounds you'll experience in those situations. In time, it does become easier.

Remember that it takes time to get accustomed to hearing with new hearing aids. Regular daily practice will help you to get the most out of your investment. The schedule in Table 4-1 can serve as a guide during the early weeks of using new hearing aids.

52. Must I Wear Them All the Time?

After the gradual adjustment period described in the previous answer, it is recommended that most hearing aid users will achieve maximum benefit from their instruments by wearing them full-time during their waking hours. You do need to remove your hearing aids when you sleep or whenever you are around water to bathe, swim, or shave.

TABLE 4-1 ···

ADJUSTING TO YOUR HEARING AIDS

Ranked from Easiest (1) to Most Difficult (11)

1. Talk in a quiet room about familiar, everyday things with a friend. One person should talk. Practice listening with the sound source in different positions and at varying distances.

2. Move to a kitchen, where acoustics are not quite so good. Listen to one person talking or to water running at different levels—just not too loud.

3. Try listening to TV in a quiet room. Choose a program that's easy to follow. Try listening to a radio or TV after it has been adjusted to a comfortable loudness level by a person with normal hearing.

4. Try to follow a conversation at a quiet dinner table.

5. Engage in conversation in a quiet room with two, then three or four, other people.

6. Move outside to a quiet place. Make it your goal to become accustomed to wind noise.

7. Walk along the street in a quiet neighborhood.

8. Attend a gathering at a church, a lecture, or a play. The first time, sit as close to the speakers as possible. The next time, try listening at a distance.

9. Try driving. Listen to the background noises. Try opening the window to listen.

10. Try a shopping trip.

11. Try to follow a conversation at a party or a restaurant or in a room where a number of people are talking. If you did not use your hearing aids constantly, they would require continuous adjustment to environmental sounds.

Because you cannot anticipate when you will need your hearing aids, the best place for them is in your ears, turned on and ready to help. Only using hearing aids for special occasions is probably one of the worst things that a hearing aid user can do. Usually, these special times are noisy and as such are possibly the worst situations for listening and communicating, even with good hearing.

Following a gradual adjustment schedule can prevent the "dresser drawer" syndrome often connected with hearing aids and allows you to get your full advantage of the instruments. Getting accustomed to your hearing aids on a regular basis prepares you for the more challenging listening experiences that we all encounter.

53. Are There Situations When a Hearing Aid Doesn't Help?

Communicating in a noisy environment is always challenging because of the interference of the noise. This is true for everyone, but it's probably more annoying for hearing aid users. Whenever possible, it is useful to reduce background noise to improve the listening situation. Some hearing aids are being manufactured with special circuits that can reduce the effects of background noise to some degree. If this is not possible, then hearing aid users may find that reducing the volume on their hearing aids tones down the level of noise they experience and allows them to concentrate on watching their communication partner's lips and facial expressions for additional help in communicating.

In an automobile, hearing aid users might try to regulate the volume control of the hearing aid that is worn on the ear next to the window. This can eliminate some of the interference of outside traffic noise.

Even though hearing aids manufactured today are technologically more and more sophisticated, they remain amplifiers of sound. Many people who use hearing aids will tell you that they find them most effective when they are used in a quiet area with one or two people speaking at a normal conversational distance. If a speaker moves away or the area becomes noisy, hearing aids become less effective. It is important that potential hearing aid users realize the limitations of mechanical hearing aids. It is also worth knowing that other technical means are available for overcoming particular everyday problems *(see Chapter 5)*.

54. Will My Voice Change when I Wear Hearing Aids?

One of the first things that all persons with new hearing aids say is that their voice sounds "different" than without the instruments. This is true since the hearing aids are amplifying all sounds, including the voice of the user. A certain amount of time, practice, and skillful volume adjustment is needed to allow hearing aid users the opportunity to get accustomed to the experience of hearing their voice differently. For most people, after regular daily practice this adjustment period is only a few days.

For some, it is useful to practice reading aloud for five to ten minutes each day. This can help you to adapt to this new experience. If you do public speaking, you should practice speaking aloud with your new hearing aids so you will be able to monitor your voice.

55. Can Hearing Aids Really Make Speech Clear?

Hearing aids can make sounds louder, which can make speech easier to hear and understand. However, the hearing aid itself cannot make speech clearer. People with a sensori-neural hearing loss and reduced speech discrimination ability may be able to hear things louder with a hearing aid, but they may still have a problem understanding each word that is being said. They may need to lipread as well to keep up with the conversation.

This can at times lead to misunderstandings because there is a tendency to think that wearing hearing aids will completely correct a hearing problem. It is useful to keep in mind that the hearing aid is simply an "aid"; for good, effective communication to be exchanged, additional assistance may need to be included. A hearing aid can improve the loss of sound intensity, but it will not restore the loss of discrimination in the ear itself.

56. What Is the T-Switch For?

The T-switch built into some hearing aids can help you hear better on the telephone as well as at group gatherings in rooms that are equipped with an audio loop system *(Question 78)* When you switch your hearing aid to "T" the microphone is disconnected and a pickup coil is activated *(see Figure 4-6)*. This tiny coil of wire picks up magnetic waves from an audio loop system or a telephone inductive coupler. You will find that environmental background noise is reduced, and once you have adjusted the volume control on your hearing aid, speech may be clearer. You may also equip your living room with a loop to help you hear better when you are watching television or talking with family and friends. Cars can also be fitted with a loop system to provide you with hearing assistance in noisy traffic.

FIGURE 4-6
A TELEPHONE SWITCH (T-SWITCH)

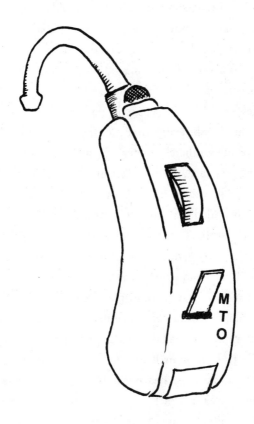

M - MICROPHONE

T - TELEPHONE

O - OFF

57. Are Hearing Aids Difficult to Care For?

It is not difficult to care for hearing aids, but they do require regular attention to keep them working at their best. Since earmolds become soiled and worn, proper care needs to be used to optimize their effectiveness. Removing the earmold from the hearing aid and washing it weekly in a gentle detergent is advisable. Using an air blower *(see Figure 4-7)*, dry the earmold well before attaching it back onto the hearing aid. The plastic tubing used to connect an earmold to a behind-the-ear hearing aid hardens and deteriorates with use and needs to be replaced on a regular basis. For some, this may be every three months, six months, or once a year; it depends on the chemistry of your body. When the earmold tubing gets hard, it affects the sound quality of the hearing aid and may also cause your hearing aid to whistle (feedback).

It is recommended that when hearing aids are not being worn, they should be stored in a small, hard-sided container with a drying agent in it to remove moisture. Dri-aid kits for this purpose can be purchased from your hearing aid dispenser *(see Figure 4-7)*, or you can make your own by placing a quarter cup of rice in a sealable plastic container. Since moisture and humidity do cause hearing aids to break down, this preventive measure is very worthwhile to keep your hearing aids working at their best.

Next, you must keep hearing aids clean of earwax. Every morning use a cleaning pick *(Figure 4-7)* to gently remove earwax from the nib opening of the hearing aid or earmold. Hold the hearing aid or earmold so that the nib faces toward the ground so that the earwax will fall out. It is best to do this in the morning since any earwax that has found its way into the nib will have hardened and will come out as a small piece. If you try to remove the earwax before it has hardened, you may accidentally push it into the hearing aid and damage the delicate components. If you did not receive a cleaning pick when you purchased your hearing aids, buy one from your dispenser Do not use a straight

FIGURE 4-7

EQUIPMENT FOR MAINTAINING HEARING AIDS

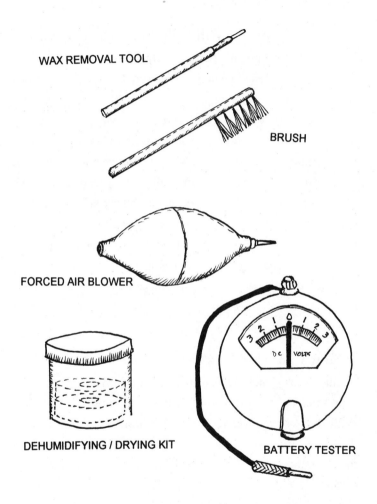

WAX REMOVAL TOOL

BRUSH

FORCED AIR BLOWER

DEHUMIDIFYING / DRYING KIT

BATTERY TESTER

pin or a toothpick; these can damage the components of your hearing aid or the tubing of your earmold.

When you take your hearing aid off at night, wipe it with a tissue to remove perspiration.

58. What Equipment Will Help Keep Them Working?

Some of the equipment that will help keep your hearing aids working well is described in the answer to the previous question. A drying agent, a cleaning pick, and an air blower are very useful. In addition, there is a moisture wrap that can be used for body-worn and behind-the-ear hearing aids to help protect them from perspiration or moisture. Special cleaning and disinfectant sprays can be obtained for cleaning the outer part of the hearing aid and/or earmold. This is especially useful if you have a history of allergies or ear infections. If you are caring for someone else's hearing aids, a battery tester and listening stethoscope are very worthwhile to purchase. Both can assist you to monitor that the hearing aid is working at its best. You can purchase a variety of equipment from your hearing aid dispenser. Some of these products are illustrated in Figure 4-7.

59. How Can a Hearing Aid Be Tested?

Because hearing aids are delicate electronic instruments, you can expect that at one time or another they may not work. There are many things that you can do to troubleshoot the instruments. See the "Look and Listen Check for Hearing Aids" *(Table 4-2)* and the "Troubleshooting Guide for Hearing Aids" *(Table 4-3)*. Check each component in the order listed. If a problem remains after you have tested the hearing aids by following these guides, schedule an appointment with your hearing aid dispenser, who has the equipment to perform a test called an *electroacoustic analysis* with a hearing aid analyzer. This test reports the function of the hearing aid, noting the amount of gain available and whether the instrument is amplifying clearly or in a distorted way.

LOOK AND LISTEN CHECK FOR HEARING AIDS

EARMOLD OR IN-THE-EAR AID
Look: Make sure the opening is clear. Look for cracks or rough areas. Check the fit.

Listen: Use sounds /a/u/ć/ʃ/s/ (pronounced *ah, oo, se, sh, s*).

BATTERY
Look: Using a battery tester, check the voltage (replace at 1.1 or below). Is the compartment clean? Are the battery contacts clean? Is the battery inserted properly? (Match + on battery to + on battery compartment.) Is the battery compartment clicked shut all the way?

CASE
Look: Check for cracks and separations.

Listen: Press the case gently. Is there an interruption in amplification?

MICROPHONE
Look: Is it clean? Is there visible damage?

DIALS
Look: Are they clean? Are they easily rotated?

Listen: Rotate the dials. Is there reasonable gain variation? Static?

SWITCHES
Look: Are they clean and easy to move?

Listen: Turn on and off. Is there static?

CORD (FOR A BODY-WORN AID)
Look: Is it cracked or frayed? Are the connection plugs clean? Are the connections tight?

Listen: Run your fingers down the cord. Is the sound clean? Is there an interruption in amplification?

TUBING (FOR A BEHIND-THE-EAR AID)
Look: Check for cracks and for a good connection to the earmold and aid. Look for moisture or debris.

Listen: Cover opening of earmold. Turn the volume to maximum gain. Do you hear feedback?

RECEIVER (FOR A BODY-WORN AID)
Look: Check for cracks. It should be firmly attached to the earmold snap.

Listen: Is there distortion or static? Reduced gain? (Substitute a spare receiver and recheck.)

VOLUME CONTROL

Look: Is there a smooth, gradual increase?

Listen: Are the five speech sounds clearly amplified?

IS THERE DISTORTION OR FEEDBACK?

Look: Recheck the receiver snap, tubing, and earmold.

Listen: Turn to maximum gain to check for internal and external feedback?

TABLE 4-3 ···

TROUBLESHOOTING GUIDE FOR HEARING AIDS

Causes	*Solutions*
"DEAD" HEARING AID (NO SOUND AT ALL)	
1. Battery dead	1. Replace battery
2. Battery + and – reversed	2. Make sure + and – are correctly placed
3. Plugs (in cord-type) broken or dirty	3. Clean or replace cord
4. Cord broken	4. Replace cord
5. Earmold or tubing plugged	5. Clean
6. Disconnected, twisted, or kinked tubing	6. Push tubing firmly onto aid or straighten tubing
7. Moisture in tubing	7. Remove moisture (use forced-air earmold cleaner)
8. Controls:	8. Check controls:
a. on-off switch	a. Make sure it is "on"
b. selector	b. Switch to "M" (microphone)
c. volume	c. Turn to appropriate setting
DISTORTION OF SOUND OR NOISY HEARING AID	
1. Battery weak	1. Replace battery
2. Contacts dirty or broken	2. Clean or replace
3. Cord broken	3. Replace
4. Poor connection between aid and earmold	4. Check connections and make adjustments
5. Volume control	5. Check volume control setting
6. Microphone opening dirty	6. Remove dirt from microphone; be sure microphone is left uncovered
7. Earmold or in-the-ear opening plugged	7. Remove wax or dirt with wax loop remover; wash earmold if needed

8. Moisture in earmold and/or tubing   8. Dry earmold and/or tubing well

9. Tubing collapsed or twisted   9. Untwist and open tubing

INTERMITTENT SOUND (AID GOES ON AND OFF)

1. Battery almost dead   1. Put in new battery

2. Bad volume switch   2. Take to hearing aid dispenser for repair

3. Moisture in tubing   3. Dry tubing (use forced-air blower)

FEEDBACK (WHISTLING NOISE)

1. Earmold not completely inserted   1. Make sure earmold fits

2. Earmold too small   2. Fit new mold

3. Tubing between aid and mold loose, broken, cracked   3. Check tubing and replace if necessary

4. Volume control turned too high   4. Turn volume down (but not below its normal setting)

5. Internal feedback inside aid due to defect in aid   5. Check with audiologist

60. Should I Insure My Hearing Aids?

Most definitely. Keep in mind that all new hearing aids have a warrantee for the first year for repairs. After the warrantee expires, there is a charge. If you are interested in obtaining insurance protection for loss, check to see if you can add a rider to your homeowner's insurance. If you would prefer to obtain coverage from an independent company, obtain information from your hearing aid dispenser about an independent company that provides a hearing instrument insurance plan protecting for loss, theft, and damage. Charges range from about $35.00 to $85.00 per year per hearing aid, depending on the type you have.

61. What Types of Hearing Aids Are Used by Children?

Children use the same types of hearing aids as adults. Hearing aids are not specifically designed for children. However, some manufacturers are now producing brightly colored instruments and earmolds that might appeal to children. Children often use supplementary listening systems, particularly in a classroom. These systems are called *assistive listening systems* or *auditory trainers.* Most schools use an FM listening system or an audio loop system for children who need hearing help in the classroom. In a noisy classroom, these systems bring the sound of the teacher's voice directly to the child, interfacing through a receiver worn in each ear or worn with an audio loop receiver around the child's neck, which interacts through the magnetic coil of each hearing aid.

The FM listening system *(Figure 4-8)* has two parts. The teacher wears a transmitter coupled to a microphone, which can be built in or attached to a cord so that it can be fixed to a shirt collar or jacket lapel. The signals from the transmitter are picked up by radio receivers worn by the student. The receiver may be part of a special hearing aid or a separate unit that can be connected to an ordinary hearing aid. The connection is often by means of an induction loop worn around the neck with the hearing aid set on the "T" position, or by a direct wire link, called *direct audio input,* if the hearing aid has a socket fitted for this purpose.

The audio loop system *(Figure 4-9)* requires that the classroom be equipped with a magnetic loop set around the periphery. When the loop is attached to an amplifier, it can be accessed by the student by switching the hearing aid to the "T" position. The teacher (or speaker) must use a microphone plugged into the amplifier.

FIGURE 4-8 ··

AN FM ASSISTIVE LISTENING SYSTEM / AUDITORY TRAINER

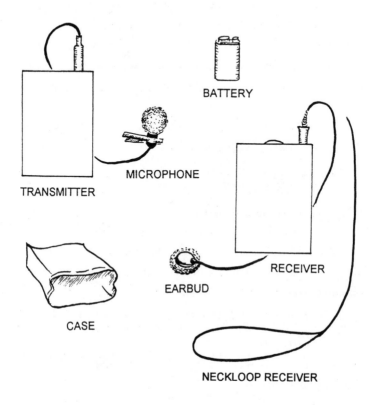

TRANSMITTER

MICROPHONE

BATTERY

RECEIVER

EARBUD

CASE

NECKLOOP RECEIVER

FIGURE 4-9 ··

AN AUDIO LOOP ASSISTIVE LISTENING SYSTEM

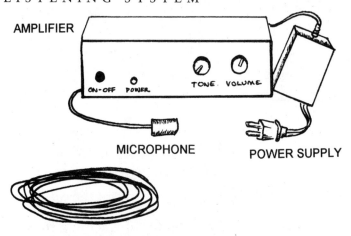

AMPLIFIER

ON-OFF POWER TONE VOLUME

MICROPHONE   POWER SUPPLY

WIRE FOR LOOP AROUND ROOM

Either system can greatly improve listening for a student who has a hearing loss. Each has its pros and cons, depending on the situation and the needs of the child.

62. How Can I Keep My Child's Hearing Aids from Falling Off?

A plastic tube that encircles the ear and attaches to the hearing aid is useful to help hold it onto your child's ear. Different manufacturers make these products. Check with the hearing aid dispenser for detailed sources. Eyeglass retainer cords can also be secured around each earhook and then pinned on your child's collar to keep them from getting lost if they do fall off the ear. You can also use clear fishing line to do the same thing. (Adults can use fishing line for their own hearing instruments if necessary.) Some parents have used two-sided cellophane tape to help keep a hearing aid in place. If your child is using body hearing aids, halters and vests can be purchased or made to hold them in place. Sport-type headbands can also be used to help to hold the hearing aid or earmold in place.

63. Why Do Hearing Aids Vary in Price and Cost So Much?

Hearing aids vary in price depending on the size, style, amount of power needed, and circuitry included. Spending more money does not always guarantee something better. It is wise to get advice from your audiologist with specific recommendations for your needs. What is best for your friend or relative may not be best for you.

Since each instrument is handcrafted specifically for the individual's needs (not mass-produced), the cost for a hearing aid can range from approximately $500 to $2000 per unit depending on the technology involved.

64. Can I Get Financial Help to Buy Hearing Aids?

If you need hearing aids and you cannot afford to purchase them, financial assistance may be available. If you are eligible for Medicaid, you should check to see if your state's Medicaid program offers assistance. If you are a veteran, you can receive a complete medical and audiological examination of your ears and hearing at one of the Veterans Administration (VA) hospitals. Check if you are eligible for free hearing aids by contacting your nearest VA hospital or regional office. You may also check with your state's vocational rehabilitation or public health departments. Some social service organizations also assist people to obtain hearing healthcare. Check with your local Lions Clubs, Sertoma Groups, or regional speech and hearing clinic for more detailed information.

65. How Else Can a Hearing Aid Help Me?

When you learn to hear with your hearing aid your speech will improve, your relationships with your spouse and family should be smoother, you will probably feel more confident on the job, you will feel more interested in socializing, and you should feel less weary and stressed since the strain of trying to hear has been reduced. The hearing aid will not solve all of your problems, but it will make everyday interactions less difficult and more comfortable.

66. Will People Be Able to See My New Hearing Aids?

Most people have concerns regarding the appearance of hearing instruments and express the worry that people will see their hearing aids. There is still a lot of misunderstanding about hearing impairment and hearing aids. But, the saying "your hearing loss is more conspicuous than your hearing aid" is really true. If you miss what others are saying, they may assume that you are not interested or that you're ignoring them. Both are worse than having them know about your hearing loss.

67. What Are Cochlear Implants?

A cochlear implant is not a transplant in which an organ is removed from the body of one person and placed into the body of another. An implant is an artificial device imbedded into the body that, through electrical stimulation of appropriate nerve endings, allows the body to function in an improved way. A cochlear implant *(Figure 3-1)* involves the surgical implantation of an electrode designed to carry electrical current into or onto the cochlea (the inner ear). The user must wear an external speech processor, which provides stimulation of the electrodes in a coded fashion. This speech processor is about the size of a small calculator and has a cord attached to a microphone that is either worn over the user's ear—just like a behind-the-ear hearing aid—or in the headpiece.

The cochlear implant is an extremely helpful device intended for persons who are profoundly hard of hearing or deaf and who receive little assistance from conventional hearing aids. They are approved by the FDA for use by children age two and older and adults. They do not restore "normal" hearing, but they do give the user an awareness of the sounds in the environment, facilitating improved lipreading ability and an improved connection with the world. Some users are able to understand speech with lipreading, others are able to understand some speech without lipreading, and some are able to understand speech on the telephone.

For more information about the cochlear implant, contact your ear, nose, and throat physician or your audiologist or call Cochlear Corporation at (800) 523-5798 (voice), (800) 483-3123 (TTY), and/or Advance Bionics at (800) 678-2575 (voice), (800) 678-3575 (TTY).

CHAPTER FIVE

Assistance Beyond the *Hearing Aid*

68. What Else Can Help?

Hearing aids can and do provide a good deal of help, but there are times when hearing aids cannot help. For example, since very few people wear a hearing aid to bed, it might be impossible for them to hear an alarm clock. Many people cannot hear the door- bell ring or a fire alarm sound if they have removed their hearing aids. Hearing clearly on the telephone or hearing a television pro- gram may be difficult for a person with a severe hearing loss, even with the best hearing aids. For these types of situations, there are devices that can provide assistance beyond the hearing aid. These are called *assistive listening devices and systems* (ALDS). An assistive listening device and system is defined as any device besides a hearing aid that is designed to improve a hearing- impaired person's ability to communicate and to function more independently despite hearing loss, either by transmitting ampli- fied sound more directly from its source to the listener—as with an induction audio loop, infrared system, FM system, or hard- wire personal communication device—or by transforming it into a tactile or visual signal. These devices can help people with hearing loss to function with greater ease in many situations of daily living. *Addresses to contact suppliers of ALDS are listed in Appendix 3.*

A hearing dog can also act as a useful pair of ears, telling you when someone is at the door or on the phone. These especially trained canines can help you to respond to various sounds around your home and in the environment. *(See Question 91.)*

69. How Can I Tell when the Telephone Rings?

If you have trouble hearing the telephone ring, you can get a simple attachment for your telephone that will change the pitch of the ring to a sound that is easier for you to hear as well as make the signal louder. You can also get devices that will activate a flashing light (a visual signal) or a fan (a tactile signal) when the phone rings. It is possible to be woken at night by a vibrator unit attached to the telephone. Portable units are available. Consult your audiologist, hearing aid dispenser, or your telephone company for more information.

70. What Can Help Me when I Talk on the Telephone?

You can get an amplified handset to attach to your telephone, or you can use an inductive coupler (a miniature induction loop) fitted into the telephone earpiece with your hearing aid switched to "T". Portable amplifiers are available. Public telephones equipped with special listening aids are marked, and those compatible with the telecoil on your hearing aids have a blue grommet attached to the cord on the receiver.

71. How Can a Deaf Person Use the Phone?

With special keyboard terminals or personal computers, people who cannot hear on the phone can type their message directly to the other party if the other person has a receiving unit. Called text telephones (TTY) or telephone devices for the deaf (TDD), the units come with printers or are portable (depending on the need of the user). You can try them at your hearing aid dispenser's assistive devices display or by contacting your telephone company. Additional sources are listed in Appendix 3.

72. Can a Deaf Person Speak to a Person with No Special Equipment over the Phone?

There's a special telephone service that lets you "talk" to anyone, anytime. It is called a relay service. Available in all 50 States 24 hours a day, 365 days a year since 1993, the Telecommunications Relay Service (TRS) allows people who are hard of hearing, deaf, or speech impaired—and who use a text telephone (TTY)—to communicate with people who use a standard telephone. A communications assistant (CA) relays the TTY input to the telephone customer and types that person's responses back to the TTY user. The Telecommunications Relay Service is reached with an 800 or other toll-free number. All relay calls remain strictly confidential as required by law, and no records of the contents of conversations are kept. Contacting the operator is free, but the actual call is billed. TTY customers may apply for special toll discounts since calls take more time. *See Appendix 5 for a listing of Telecommunications Relay Services in the United States.*

73. How Can I Hear Someone at the Door?

This is a common problem, especially if you live alone. It is possible to hook up a bell with a different tone or with a longer-playing melody so that it will include some tones that you can hear better than some others. You can put an extension bell or buzzer in the room you use most often. If you cannot hear these special bells, chimes, and buzzers, there are special flashing lights that can be attached to the doorbell to attract your attention. Some are portable and others must be plugged in, but you can usually accomplish installation on your own. A wristband with a vibrator attached can be used to let you "feel" when someone is at the door. All of these devices are available through catalog order supply houses. See Appendix 3 for a list of merchandisers who can send you catalogs.

74. What Can I Use to Help Wake Me Up?

Conventional alarm clocks can produce a variety of signals to awaken you. It is worth trying different models to check which one you hear best. Often, getting a clock radio and tuning it to a newscaster will help because most people can usually hear a speaker's voice easier than a high-pitched bell. There are a wide variety of vibrating alarm clocks, some that shake the pillow and others strong enough to shake the mattress. Other special alarms can be connected to a lamp that will flash or a fan that will swirl and awaken you. Some are small, compact, and battery-operated, which makes them perfect for traveling. Test them out at a demonstration center of assistive devices.

75. Are There Special Fire and Smoke Alarms?

Alarms that will cause a light to flash, a receiver to vibrate, or a fan to circulate can be set up so that you can see or feel if a fire emergency occurs. There are many different types of systems that can be hooked up in a simple manner to make your home, office, or hotel/motel room safer. You will see several types of alerting systems listed in assistive devices catalogs *(see Appendix 3)*. In addition, you can contact an alarm and safety supply facility in your area to inquire about special fire and smoke alarm systems for people who have difficulty hearing the standard whistle or bell. This is critical for your safety.

76. How Can I Hear My Baby Cry?

It can be very troublesome if your hearing impairment prevents you from hearing your baby cry. There are, however, several varieties of a simple alerting system that will help. This type of baby alarm uses a flashing light or a vibrating wrist-worn receiver to attract your attention when the baby cries. It is also possible to get a vibrating disc or pad to put under your pillow or mattress if you feel that a light will not work for you at night. Baby cry systems can be found in the catalogs and tried at an assistive devices center. There are also standard baby monitors available at most department stores and infant shops.

77. What Can I Use to Hear the Television More Easily?

Many TVs are fitted with sockets into which you can plug headphones or a special TV listening aid. You can have your television repair person install such a socket if yours doesn't come with one. It can be set up with a switch that can be set to allow only the person with the earphones audibility to hear or switched to include the others in the room. Many headphones are available of varying quality and price. It is a good idea to test out the product to be certain of its quality and usefulness for your listening needs.

If your hearing loss is more severe, you may find a TV listening aid helpful. Several are available and can be plugged directly into the TV set, while others pick up the sound with a small microphone set near the speaker of the television set. These systems are useful if your TV does not have an earphone socket.

A TV band radio is not expensive and is useful when placed near your ear to bring the sound closer and make it more audible. You could also use an induction audio loop around your chair so that you could listen through your own hearing aid set at "T" and/or use a closed caption circuit *(see Questions 78 and 82)*.

78. What Is an Induction Audio Loop?

As illustrated in Figure 4-9, the induction audio loop system is used in conjunction with a hearing aid's telephone switch. The loop is connected to a special amplifier that receives the signal from the sound source. It works on the simple principle that when an electric current passes through a wire, it produces a magnetic field around that wire. When the wire is formed into a loop, a magnetic field is produced throughout the area enclosed by the loop. The loop system is useful for groups of all sizes and miniature systems can be installed in your home to enhance TV listening or in your car to improve your ability to hear above the noise of the car (the signal-to-noise ratio) as you are driving.

The loop can be big enough to cover the interior of a cathedral or small enough to be used with the telephone receiver, provided that there is an adequate level of current flowing in the wire so a satisfactory level of magnetic field results. The magnetic field can be picked up by a small coil of wire built into many hearing aids. The coil is selected by moving the switch to the marked "T" (telephone) position. The hearing aid then converts the magnetic field back into sound for the user to hear. The biggest advantage of the loop system is that the owner of a hearing aid equipped with a telephone coil already has half of the system.

79. What Is an Infrared System?

An infrared listening system consists of a transmitter *(Figure 5-1)* and a receiver *(Figure 5-2);* the medium is invisible light. The transmitter emits a signal consisting of light waves, which spread throughout the room. The wavelength of the light is outside the range of what humans can see. These light waves carry the message from the sound source and are picked up by receivers worn by the user. A stethoscope earphone can be used, as can the infrared receiver coupled to the user's own hearing aid telephone coil. Infrared systems are wireless and offer excellent fidelity for radio, TV, stereo concerts, lectures, and theater. Due to the light-based principle of operation, however, infrared signals must be contained within the physical confines of the space in which the transmitters are installed.

FIGURE 5-1

AN INFRARED ASSISTIVE LISTENING SYSTEM

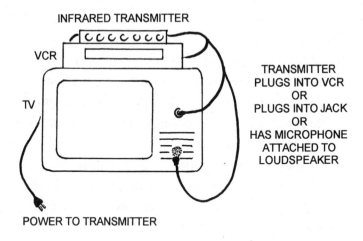

INFRARED TRANSMITTER

VCR

TV

TRANSMITTER
PLUGS INTO VCR
OR
PLUGS INTO JACK
OR
HAS MICROPHONE
ATTACHED TO
LOUDSPEAKER

POWER TO TRANSMITTER

FIGURE 5-2

INFRARED RECEIVERS

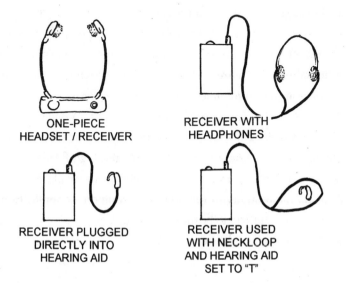

ONE-PIECE
HEADSET / RECEIVER

RECEIVER WITH
HEADPHONES

RECEIVER PLUGGED
DIRECTLY INTO
HEARING AID

RECEIVER USED
WITH NECKLOOP
AND HEARING AID
SET TO "T"

80. What Is an FM System?

The FM system shown in Figure 4-8 is a radio system consisting of a small transmitter and a receiver. The transmitter microphone is placed near the sound source, and a signal is sent to the receiver. The receiver picks up the signal and sends the sound into the user's ears by way of some type of earphone receiver. A variation of this system consists of a receiver with a wire loop worn around the neck. The wire acts as an antenna and is connected to the receiver. The neck loop transmits the signal to hearing aids that are switched to the "T" position (this position makes the hearing aids sensitive to the magnetic field generated by the wire). The FM system is wireless, offers excellent fidelity for all communication and listening situations, and is generally free of interference. The user may also move anywhere within the transmitting range of the system and receive high-quality signals from the source.

81. What Is a Hardwire Personal Communicator?

The hardwire personal system is designed to bring the listener closer to the source of the desired sound, thus reducing undesirable background noise and providing greater intelligibility. The hardwire system is so named because the user is connected directly to an immobile electronic system by an earphone or headphones *(see Figure 5-3)*. The hardwire systems are excellent for one-on-one communication such as interviews and counseling sessions, in a car, in small groups, and for TV viewing and radio and stereo enjoyment. Hardwire systems offer good sound quality since minimal signal loss occurs and high-fidelity headsets can be used. As a wire system, however, it may place limitations on the mobility of the user depending on its application. Such systems are said to be the simplest and least expensive of the four types of assistive listening systems.

FIGURE 5-3 ···

A HARDWIRE ASSISTIVE LISTENING SYSTEM

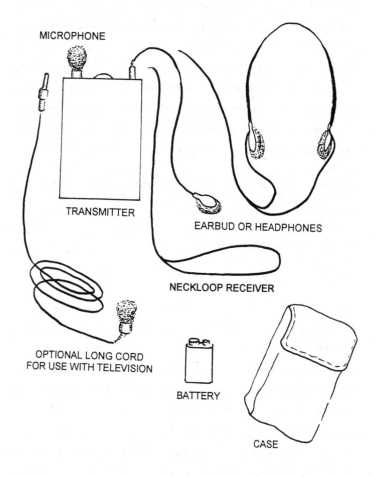

MICROPHONE

TRANSMITTER

EARBUD OR HEADPHONES

NECKLOOP RECEIVER

OPTIONAL LONG CORD
FOR USE WITH TELEVISION

BATTERY

CASE

82. Would Closed Caption (CC) Television Help Me?

Closed Caption television transmits the dialogue and information on the TV screen in a printed format that is similar to subtitles. You can only see the printed format if you have a television with closed captioning capability (all televisions built after July 1993) or if you have a separate closed caption decoder. These subtitles can be of great assistance if you have hearing difficulties. Television programs that are captioned are marked with "CC" in the TV listings. Many videos are available with this feature as well.

83. What Can Be Done to Help Me Hear While at My Job?

If you need help hearing on the telephone, there are many different types of amplifiers that can be built into your work phone or added on. Speak with the telephone installation personnel or your supervisor to investigate which system would work best for you.

If you have a secretary, have this person help you by identifying who is calling; knowing who the person is makes it easier to anticipate their message and understand. You may also use an answering machine to first screen your calls; this will allow you time to prepare for the conversation.

A flashing light can be installed to signal when the phone is ringing. If needed, a text telephone (TTY) can be made available. Flashing lights can also be installed to signal when a customer enters a shop or when the fire or smoke alarm goes off. For greater ease at meetings, an assistive listening device (described in Questions 78 through 81) could be very helpful to assure that you don't miss important information.

You will find it helpful to coordinate your schedule to pace the demands on your hearing. If you have to be in meetings in the morning, try to arrange for a quieter afternoon of paperwork. If you are in meetings all day, give yourself time to rest when you arrive home. Hearing is very hard work, and it is not unusual for you to be weary after a day of listening on the job.

84. What Can Help Me to Hear at Plays and Movies?

The Americans with Disabilities Act (ADA) mandates that theaters that feature live productions and films make their programs accessible to people with hearing loss. Most have installed FM or infrared assistive listening systems. Ask at the ticket window how you can borrow a unit for help with hearing while attending a program. There is usually no charge, but a deposit of cash, a credit card, or a driver's license is often asked for and held until after the show when you return the receiving unit.

85. How Can I Hear Better in a Church or Temple?

If a house of worship is to minister effectively to all of its members, including persons with hearing loss, the facility must be accessible. Be an advocate for yourself and all of the others in your church community who do not hear well. Share information with your minister or rabbi about assistive listening devices. Many churches and temples have installed special supplementary listening systems for use during services. They can either be integrated with the sound system in use or be used separately. Demonstrate their function and encourage their use. Appoint a committee to keep them working properly.

86. What Is a Total Access Courtroom?

If you are called to jury duty but you have difficulty hearing, it is possible to take advantage of real-time reporting technology. A court reporter operating the Computer-Aided Transcription (CAT) system allows the stenographer to be linked electronically to a computer, instantly translating the court reporter's electronic signals into English. Once captured by the computer, this information can be provided in the form best suited to each individual's needs: to a laptop, in Braille, or as real-time text or captions for hearing-impaired or deaf persons. By integrating video with CAT, court reporters can transmit real-time captions to monitors strategically placed throughout the courtroom. As the proceedings are recorded by the court reporter and on video-tape, the CAT system synchronizes the English text with the video. The judge or attorneys can retrieve both the text and video portions of the testimony for review as well. For further information, contact the

NATIONAL COURT REPORTERS ASSOCIATION
8224 Old Courthouse Road
Vienna, VA 22182
(703) 556-6272 (voice)
(703) 556-6289 (TTY)

Work with the court personnel in your community to make them aware of TAC capabilities.

87. Is It Possible for Me to Try These Devices and Systems?

See if your audiologist has devices and systems for you to try. Throughout the United States, centers are available where you can try out many of the assistive listening devices and systems, determine what is useful for your communication and listening needs, and receive information about where you can purchase what you need. Check with your audiologist or hearing aid dispenser to locate the nearest center to you.

88. Where Can I Buy Assistive Devices and Systems?

Some audiologists and hearing aid dispensers have assistive devices and systems available for demonstration, trial, and purchase, as do some telephone companies. Check in your community. You will also find a list of merchandisers who have catalogs available in Appendix 3.

89. What General Tips Can Teachers Follow to Help Students Hear Better in the Classroom?

These general tips for teachers can improve learning in the classroom for the student with hearing loss. Share them with your child's teachers.

1. Provide instructions or a written agenda or lesson plan on the board or as a handout.

2. Seat the student near the teacher or speaker.

3. Arrange for a note taker in class, or a copy of the teacher's notes if a note taker is not available.

4. Administer written tests instead of oral tests.

5. Use an assistive listening device (e.g., FM system) if recommended.

6. Be aware that oral, sign language, or cued speech interpreters are available and call on their services.

7. Provide one-on-one testing for oral exams (e.g., spelling tests, vocabulary tests, and foreign language tests).

Remember that two students with almost identical hearing problems may function very differently and can therefore not be lumped into a generalized category. The age of onset, social maturity, family background, and support and intelligence are factors affecting a student's ability to function.

90. What Specific Suggestions for Teachers Can Help Students with a Hearing Loss?

These specific suggestions for teachers can improve the student's learning experience. Share them with your child's teacher.

1. Preferential seating is important. It includes placing the student with the best ear toward the speaker, as well as seating the student within six feet of the speaker. Since the focus of attention

may change during a lecture, the student should be assured that any change of seat will not be considered disruptive.

2. The speaker should face the student when speaking so that lip movements, gestures, and facial expressions can be seen. Make sure the lighting is on the speaker and not in the student's eyes. The student must be able to maintain full view of the speaker's face during the presentation of lessons. The speaker should avoid talking without facing the class (e.g., when writing on the blackboard); standing in front of a window or bright light; teaching from the back of the room where the student cannot see; and walking around the classroom while talking.

3. The speaker should choose a careful, yet natural, manner and avoid exaggerated lip movements.

4. When speakers address a hearing-impaired student, they should make sure the student is attending and then speak.

5. The speaker should rephrase (rather than repeat) statements that are not initially understood.

6. It is helpful to inform the student in advance what material will be covered on a particular day so that pertinent material can be read in advance.

7. Use visual aids/media (e.g., the blackboard or an overhead projector) to supplement spoken information in lessons. When using films or movies, try to obtain a captioned film. If that's not possible, obtain a written transcript. When written material must be copied by the student, lecturing should not occur at the same time.

8. It is difficult for the hearing-impaired student to use visual clues (such as speechreading) in class and take notes simultaneously. Special lecture notes or notes shared by a fellow student or a note taker may be helpful.

9. Oral tests should be avoided because they can be penalizing to the hearing-impaired student.

10. The student may not be able to hear loudspeaker announcements. The teacher or a fellow student should keep the hearing-impaired student aware of any important messages.

11. A student's ability to hear may fluctuate. Straining or watching intently to understand through speechreading, as well as the strain to listen, may make the student tire easily. Allow periodic time for hearing-impaired students to rest their eyes and relax.

12. Take steps to improve the signal-to-noise ratio. Install sound-absorbing surfaces such as carpeting or corkboard and use FM systems coupled to the student's hearing aids.

13. Encourage your students by using the following communication strategies:

Help the children to make it a habit to watch speakers even if listening is not difficult. It is good to get in the habit of paying attention.

Teach the children not to interrupt speakers before they finish a sentence. The children may not understand the beginning, but may catch the end.

Instruct the children to let speakers know if something that was said was missed and to ask for it to be repeated.

Face the children when speaking and use normal speech. A hearing-impaired individual needs to have a clear view of your face. Exaggerated mouth movements and overly emphasized speech can make speechreading more difficult. Distance, bright light behind the speaker, heavy mustaches, and accents can make speechreading difficult. Also, remember that things you say with your back turned while writing on the chalkboard will not be heard or understood. If the children do not understand you, try repeating and slowing down. If repeating doesn't work, try rephrasing what you have said in language that's more familiar to the children.

Help the children learn to summarize what they did hear so that the communication partner knows what to fill in.

Identify the topic being discussed. When listeners know what a person is talking about, it is easier to follow the conversation.

Help students learn to look for ideas rather than isolated words.

Guide students to keep alert for key words in sentences in order to follow ideas.

Using the clues from the situation helps listeners to get meanings. Teach students that the idea is often spelled out by the actual situation. They may be able to anticipate words or phrases that will probably be used.

Tell students not to be afraid to guess using situational and contextual clues.

Teach the students to keep informed of friends' interests. If they and their friends have favorite topics, this known limited content makes understanding easier.

Encourage students to ask friends to help keep them informed about things that are happening in school (e.g., announcements over the loud speaker), in their community, and in their neighborhood, and about events in the lives of people they know.

Help students with hearing loss to understand that they may feel more fatigue after classes since they must work so much harder to keep up with the information presented.

Accept the hearing-impaired children positively since your attitudes and feelings are reflected in the behaviors of the other children and affect how the children feel about themselves.

Remember that the hearing-impaired children are children first, with their own strengths and needs. Every child needs to gain confidence by doing things well, and each requires support in areas of need.

Encourage speech. Hearing-impaired children should have developed some speech ability before being placed in your classroom. Activities in your class can help improve their speech development because of the strong need to be understood by hearing classmates. Encourage and reinforce talking. Give the children opportunities to speak with you and with the other children. Ask the children to repeat or rephrase what is said if you don't understand. Don't pretend to understand if you don't. Don't interrupt the children to make constant speech corrections. Teach the children to use the dictionary for pronunciation, and use diacritical markings and accent marks to show correct pronunciation. Work closely with the speech clinician to reinforce specific speech skills being developed in therapy.

Explain hearing loss to the other children in the classroom. The normally hearing children in the class may have questions about the hearing aids and about the children with a hearing loss. Answer their questions directly, in a matter-of-fact way. This will demonstrate your comfort and help them accept their hearing-impaired peers.

Determine the best seating arrangement. The children and audiologist will be able to help you determine where the hearing-impaired children should sit for best listening and speech-reading advantage. If you move around the room as you teach, allow the students to move to another desk. During group discussions, the hearing-impaired students will need to turn around to follow comments from classmates. Mention the name of the student who is speaking so the hearing-impaired students can quickly find the speaker.

Remember that distance makes listening more difficult. Hearing-impaired students wearing personal hearing aids will have difficulty in understanding what is said if they are more than a few feet away from the speaker. If the students are using special auditory amplification equipment, the distance problem is reduced. During directed teaching, the students who rely on "looking and listening" will do best when seated close to you, but not so close that they must look up to see your face. Small group activities are better for listening.

Assign a student helper for each hearing-impaired student. Responsible peers or "buddies" sit nearby and clue the hearing-impaired students to page numbers, directions, and requests. Such help should be as unobtrusive as possible.

Present information visually whenever possible. Do not rely solely on oral presentation of information at the elementary level. The same outlines, schedules, assignments, and directions that you write on the board for all of your students are especially important to the hearing-impaired children. Use of transparencies, slides, charts, pictures, and other mediated materials is effective for all learners. As you get to know your hearing-impaired students, you will be able to detect that they are confused by oral directions. A quick check after the class has begun working may save the hearing-impaired children from completing the assignment incorrectly. Ask the children to repeat your directions.

Be aware of special language needs. Show the children you want to communicate with them and that you are glad to share an experience. Reinforce attempts to express ideas and feelings. Even with linguistic errors, an imaginative and enthusiastic expression is more desirable than a memorized one with little relevance or meaning. Give special emphasis to teaching word meanings, idioms, meanings conveyed by intonation, question forms, sentence structure, inferences, and conclusions. Model the children's language by responding to the incomplete thoughts or phrases with complete sentences.

Teach dictionary use. Give special attention to presentation of new vocabulary and comprehension of concepts. Relate new concepts to real experiences. In certain subjects such as science and social studies, new vocabulary is introduced rapidly. The hearing-impaired students may need extra help in learning the concepts underlying new words. Write new words on the board and have the students keep a list of new words and their meanings. Ask the teacher of the hearing-impaired, the parents, and the buddies to help reinforce new vocabulary. The hearing-impaired students may have been taught all of the words they know. They probably have not had the luxury of learning new vocabulary just by overhearing it. Make a note of idioms and words with multiple meanings and ask for help in teaching them. Work closely with the teacher of the hearing-impaired or speech-language pathologist to reinforce specific language concepts. Try to pinpoint problems and let the specialist know. Understand that communication is a complicated process involving receptive, expressive, and cognitive language processing.

Help the students develop responsibility. Hearing-impaired children need empathy, not sympathy. Classroom rules and limits must apply to them just as they apply to everyone. Assign jobs and expect responsible behavior. Ask the hearing-impaired children to tell you what the rules are, what the assignment is, or what you are requesting. Once it's understood, let them know that you expect the appropriate response or behavior from everyone. Encourage them to do errands for you, such as taking messages to the office. Give them opportunities to learn to communicate with different people in different situations (e.g., handling the lunch order or delivering materials). Show your confidence in their ability to do the job. Praise the children, as you would any child, for a job well done.

Keep in mind that concentrated looking and listening is tiring. It's hard work to sit and concentrate all day long. Remember how tired you get after a day's inservice or workshop. The hearing-impaired children sitting in your classroom for hours each day have a doubly difficult job. They have to constantly put together what is seen with what is heard, making the best guess based on situational clues and on what makes the most sense linguistically. This is part of the impact of hearing impairment, and the children need your understanding. Scheduling breaks or periods of less directed instruction may be helpful.

Include parents as part of the teaching team. Keep in close communication with the parents. Supportive parents can help contribute significantly to the children's success. Set up lines of communication with them, and let them know you are interested in their input. Welcome parents to observe their children in your classroom and let them know that you are available to them for questions and conferences. Try to alert them to problems the children may be having and work with them to solve problems that arise. The educational success of any child is affected by the degree and type of parental support given to the program. This is especially true for the hearing-impaired children in mainstream classrooms.

91. How Can I Get a Hearing Dog?

Canine helpers include guide dogs for blind persons, service dogs for people in wheelchairs, therapy dogs for the physically or emotionally disabled, and hearing dogs for people with hearing impairment. Hearing dogs assist hard of hearing or deaf individuals in coping with some of the practical difficulties of hearing loss. They assist with skills necessary for independent living and enhance the emotional lives of the owners in many ways.

Hearing dogs are trained to respond to various sounds and then alert their owners, leading them to the source of the sound. Different responses are taught for varying sound sources. A hearing dog provides another pair of ears in the house and, consequently, an increased awareness, fostering independence, providing more security, and helping to relieve anxiety. Contact the following organizations for further information:

DELTA SOCIETY
National Service Dog Center
289 Perimeter Road East
Renton, WA 98055
(800) 869-6898 (voice)
(800) 809-2714 (TTY)

CANINE WORKING COMPANIONS, INC.
RD #2 Box 170
Waterville, NY 13480
(315) 861-7770 (voice)

RED ACRE FARM HEARING DOG CENTER
Box 278, 109 Red Acre Road
Stow, MA 01775
(508) 897-8343 (voice/TTY)

DOGS FOR THE DEAF
10175 Wheeler Road
Central Point, OR 97502
(541) 826-9220 (voice/TTY)

INTERNATIONAL HEARING DOG, INC.
5901 East 89th
Henderson, CO 80640
(303) 287-3277 (voice/TTY)

92. What Can I Request To Help Me Hear Better During a Hospital Stay?

A hospital stay can be frightening, especially if you have difficulty hearing. Be certain to inform the admissions clerk when you check in and ask that the International Symbol for Hearing Impairment *(Figure 5-4)* is placed on your chart, on your wristband, above your bed, and on your door as a reminder for all staff that you need special help to hear. Remind all staff that you hear better if they face you in good light and eliminate background noise whenever possible. Advise them to always include you in the communication since the information is vital to your health and you need to know. Request an assistive listening device or an interpreter for all complex communications. Ask for an amplified receiver or TTY for the telephone in your room. Request a closed caption decoder for the television and an alerting device for a smoke or fire alarm. For additional information about a hospital access program, contact Self Help for Hard of Hearing People, Inc. (SHHH) *(See Question 108).*

FIGURE 5-4 ··

THE INTERNATIONAL SYMBOL OF ACCESS FOR PEOPLE WHO ARE DEAF AND HARD OF HEARING

93. What Can Help Me when I Travel?

In a hotel or motel, you may request alerting devices that flash a light or vibrate for the alarm clock, telephone, smoke and fire alarm, and door knock. A closed captioning device for the television or an assistive listening device can be reserved as well as a TTY or amplifier for telephone use. Make your requests when reservations are placed to assure availability.

Airplanes are noisy, so it is a good idea to request a seat near the front of the plane as far from the engines as possible. Alert the flight attendant if your hearing loss is severe enough to prevent you from hearing announcements. Airplane takeoffs and landings are difficult for some people's ears. Your physician may recommend a decongestant to be taken about an hour before takeoff. There are plugs for your ears that are designed to equalize the pressure that builds up on takeoffs and landings. They are available in sizes suitable for adults and children. Check with your dispenser, physician, or drugstore for this product. Chewing gum, yawning, or sucking on hard candy will also help to equalize the pressure in your ears. If you are wearing your hearing aids, you may want to loosen them slightly to help.

It's a good idea to allow yourself enough time to find your destination at airports. If you cannot understand the announcements over the public address system, double-check with an attendant at the gate or check with a fellow traveler. When you ask for directions, repeat what you think you heard to confirm that you understood correctly. Always carry extra batteries so you won't be caught without them when traveling.

94. Are There Music Recordings for People Who Do Not Hear Well?

Music For All To Hear, Inc. has produced music especially arranged and acoustically prepared for people with hearing loss. Holiday and Broadway recordings as well as music for children are available from:

MUSIC FOR ALL TO HEAR, INC.
PO Box 6347
Evanston, IL 60204
(708) 475-6336 (voice)

95. What Is the Emergency Alert System?

Formerly the Emergency Broadcast System, the Federal Communications Commission (FCC) has approved a new system for emergency broadcasts called the Emergency Alert System. From July 1996, all television and radio stations must comply by transmitting emergency messages in both audio and text mode, and emergency screen crawls are not to interfere with any other text messages simultaneously displayed on the screen. Cable companies must designate a specific channel for broadcast of emergency information.

CHAPTER SIX

What Else Can I Do?

96. Can I Learn to Read Lips?

We all read lips to some degree, and if you have some trouble hearing, either temporary or permanent, you'll find yourself watching the speaker more attentively to get the message. Think of times when you've been at a noisy party and how you had to concentrate on your communication partner's face. As your hearing problem increases, so does your need to pay close attention and watch the speaker for more information. We get important clues of what people are saying by watching their expression, gestures, and body language as well as their lips. If you sign up to take a lipreading (also called *speechreading*) class, you will learn how to place yourself in the best position to lipread and how to use the various clues to understand what is being said. Since it is possible to actually see only about 50 percent of the words in the English language, even the best lipreaders must rely on other cues to help understanding. Lipreading or speechreading classes will review strategies that you can use to improve your communication and listening abilities.

Table 6-1 outlines sounds to look for when lipreading and lists the visibility of different consonant sounds.

TABLE 6-1 ··

SOUNDS TO LOOK FOR WHEN SPEECHREADING

Sound	Lip Movement	Examples
MOST VISIBLE SOUNDS		
P, B	Lips pressed together	people, pull, belong, boy
M, W	Lips are rounded with small opening in center	many, more, went, we, water
WH, F, V	Upper teeth touch lower lip	what, why, when, face, four, foot, voice, vote, vacuum
SH	Lips are slightly rounded and pushed outward	shoe, shop, ship
CH, TH	Tongue is visible between the teeth	cheese, chap, church, thumb, thorn, think, three
LESS VISIBLE SOUNDS		
K, G	Tongue and soft palate	kick, kiss, give
L	Tongue and teeth	love, leaf, lady
S, Z	Tongue	sea, sun, zebra
T, D, N	Tongue	toe, dog, new

Practicing this skill will help you to take full advantage of visual clues. Read the words in the example column aloud in front of a mirror and note the differences in the movements seen on the lips for each of the sounds. You can use the words in sentences and observe how easy it is to recognize some (for example, *people*), and how difficult it is to see others (such as *kick* or *new*). It is very useful to practice lipreading with a friend or spouse.

Helping others to realize that some sounds are more difficult to see on the lips could assist them in avoiding words beginning with the less visible sounds and, whenever possible, substituting words with similar meanings that use the more visible consonants. For example, the word *dog* is very difficult to lipread, but the word *puppy* is easier to see.

97. How Can Observing the Gestures and Facial Expressions of Others when Communicating Help?

Watch gestures and facial expressions in combination with watching the lip movements of the speaker. All can convey much information and help you to understand the conversation. Examples of gestures and how we interpret them are listed in Table 6-2 so that you can practice this additional strategy to improve your communication ability.

TABLE 6-2

GESTURES AND FACIAL EXPRESSIONS

Gesture	Interpretation
COMMANDS	
Palm of hand raised to another person	Stop
Forefinger held to closed lips	Quiet
Wiggling crooked index finger	Come here
Both hands with palms open, extended forward	Stand up
Both hands with palms open, lifted two or three times	Get up
Right hand, palm open, swept forward in a pushing away gesture	Take it away; go away
Hand swept forward in a pushing away gesture	I don't want it; don't give it to me
REQUESTS	
Both arms extended, open palms turned up	Help me
Wiggling thumb and two fingers of right hand	Pay me
If fingers rubbed to palm with hand extended	Hand it to me
Hands together, palms facing in	Please
Exposing watch and looking at other person with raised eyebrows	What's the time?

Gesture	Interpretation
Bringing right hand to mouth in gesture of lifting a glass	May I have a drink?

APPROVAL OR DISAPPROVAL

Head nodding up and down	Yes; right
Head shaking sideways	No; wrong
Hands extended, palms down, moved back and forth to show reverse sides	Mediocre
Open palms brought together lightly in a clapping gesture	Good for you
Thumbs both hands down	No good

98. What Is Auditory Training?

The main purpose of auditory training is to teach you to make the best use of your remaining hearing. Amplification is provided either with your own personal hearing aids or with an auditory training unit. Auditory training sessions are often run in conjunction with hearing aid orientation classes or with lipreading classes.

99. How Can Communication Strategies Help?

Communication strategies are practical tips that can help to facilitate effective communication by giving you some techniques that make communication easier. Try to practice these in each interaction.

1.   Make it a habit to watch speakers even if listening is not difficult. It is good to get in the habit of paying attention.

2.   Don't interrupt speakers before they finish a sentence. You may not understand the beginning but may catch the end.

3.   When you are aware that you missed something that was said, ask for it to be repeated.

4.   Summarize what you did hear so that your communication partner knows what to fill in.

5. Learn the topic being discussed. When you know what a person is talking about, it is easier to follow the conversation.

6. Learn to look for ideas rather than isolated words.

7. Keep alert for key words in sentences in order to follow ideas.

8. Use the clues from the situation to help get meanings. The idea is often spelled out by the actual situation. You may be able to anticipate words or phrases that will probably be used.

9. Don't be afraid to guess using situational and contextual clues.

10. Keep informed of your friends' interests. If you and your friends have favorite topics, this limited content makes understanding easier.

11. Stay aware of current events. When you know something about a topic you can more readily recognize key words, names, and so forth. Read the daily newspaper and be aware of the programs that many people watch, even if you don't watch TV.

12. Ask family members to keep you informed about things that are happening in your community and neighborhood and about events in the lives of people you know.

13. Keep your sense of humor.

100. How Can I Improve My Listening Skills?

Improving listening skills is especially useful for a person who has experienced a hearing loss. Being attentive and paying attention is the first thing you need to do. Resist distraction. Judge the content of what is being said, not the delivery. Listen for ideas, not for each word. A good listener works hard, exhibits an active body state, listens between the lines to the tone of voice, and attends to the speaker's facial expression, gestures, body language, and other situational cues.

These specific listening tips can help:

1. Relearn the trick of concentration. Pay attention. Listen.

2. Avoid pretending that you have understood what was said. It will only confuse things later.

3. Don't be afraid to ask people to repeat or speak up louder.

4. Don't hesitate to inform speakers that you have a hearing impairment and suggest what they can do to help you hear better.

5. Remind people to speak *to* you.

6. Carefully watch the speaker. Attend to the lips, facial expressions and gestures, and body language.

7. Position yourself to take advantage of good lighting. Have the light come from behind you. Rearrange your position if you find that there is a glare on the speaker's face. This will assist you in using all nonverbal clues.

8. At informal gatherings, try to limit the number of people you speak with at one time. One-on-one conversations are easier than group conversations.

9. Hearing in noisy places is a problem for all listeners. Practice listening at parties, meetings, theaters, movies, and churches. This will help you learn to separate speech from background noise.

10. Encourage the use of public address systems at meetings or at churches when they are available.

11. Try to arrive early at large group functions so that you can have the option of sitting close to the speakers. Position yourself in the best situation to hear as well as to see.

12. Use the "T" switch when listening on the telephone, and place the receiver close to the microphone.

101. What Is Cued Speech?

Cued Speech is a system of communication developed by Dr. Orin Cornett in 1966 at Gallaudet University. It combines a manual element (the cues) with spoken language. Using the cues as well as the visual elements of speech (lipreading) helps to make the spoken word more recognizable for persons with hearing loss.

Eight different hand shapes give an indication as to which consonant is being used. Vowel sounds are shown by the position of the hand, at the corner of the mouth, at the side of the face, at the throat, or at the chin. Phonetically based, Cued Speech is a handy tool to clarify speech, and the basics can be learned in ten to twenty hours. It is not a method or a language.

For further information or for a facility near you that teaches cued speech, contact the following:

NATIONAL CUED SPEECH ASSOCIATION
PO Box 31345
Raleigh, NC 27622
(919) 828-1218 (voice)

DEPARTMENT OF AUDIOLOGY
Gallaudet University, MTB 217
800 Florida Avenue, NE
Washington, DC 20002
(202) 651-5330 (voice)

102. Is Sign Language for Me?

When most of us refer to sign language, we are talking about American Sign Language (ASL), the language of the deaf. Linguistic authorities have studied ASL and determined that it is an independent language from English. ASL is governed by its own set of grammar and syntax, has its own slang expressions, and has an expressive vocabulary numbering in the thousands. Becoming fluent in ASL is as challenging as fluently mastering any foreign language. In addition to ASL (which is the only sign language that is a language unto itself), there are several additional ways of signing. Signed English; Signing Essential English (SEE1), which involves translating grammatical English into Sign; and Signing Exact English (SEE 2), which involves a word for word verbatim translation of English into Sign, were created by educators in the 1970s to help teach English to deaf students. Pidgin Signed English (PSE) is a combination of ASL and Signed English. Signs can vary according to the method of Sign, just as differences in dialect can occur in the northern and southern regions of a country.

If you want to pursue the study of sign language, contact colleges, libraries, and regional learning centers in your area.

103. How Can an Interpreter Help?

Sign language interpreters can be hired to interpret for deaf individuals when they attend appointments, religious services, or theater events. The role of the interpreter is to translate the exchange of information to facilitate the deaf person's understanding. Interpreters must complete an extensive training curriculum and be certified to function in this capacity. In addition to sign language interpreters, oral interpreters can provide a clear, visual representation of the communication on the lips, providing the person who has difficulty hearing with the opportunity to lipread the information. To obtain a list of registered interpreters in your area, write to:

REGISTRY OF INTERPRETERS FOR THE DEAF
PO Box 1339
Washington, DC 20013

104. What Can Others Do to Help?

Our ability to communicate is strongly influenced by what other people do and how they speak. Lipreading is not possible if speakers stand against the light with their faces in a shadow, or speak while eating or with a cigarette in their mouth.

The speaker should face the listener directly in good light to facilitate communication, speaking a bit slower than usual, but not shouting. Shouting distorts the facial features and is not helpful. The speaker should speak clearly, eliminating extra words. Flip remarks and asides can be very confusing to a person who has difficulty hearing since they are difficult to follow.

It helps if others understand the communication problems of those with hearing impairment. It is important to keep in mind that carrying on a conversation in the presence of background noise is far more challenging if a person has a hearing loss. If the topic of a conversation is suddenly switched, it can be very difficult to follow.

Remember to use the following tips when communicating with a person who has difficulty hearing:

1. If necessary, speak a bit louder, but don't shout.

2. Speak clearly and slowly.

3. Speak at a distance of between three and six feet, or use an FM auditory enhancement system. Rearrange the room if necessary.

4. Stand in clear light, facing the person with whom you are speaking for greater visibility of lip movements, facial expressions, and gestures. Rearrange the room if necessary.

5. Do not speak unless your face is visible. Remember the rule, "If listeners can't see me, then they can't hear me."

6. Reduce or move away from background noise.

7. If listeners do not appear to understand what is being said, rephrase the statement rather than simply repeating the misunderstood words.

8. Do not overarticulate. Overarticulation not only distorts the sounds of speech but also distorts the speaker's face, making the use of visual clues more difficult.

9. Do not obscure your mouth with a cigarette or your hands, and do not chew food while speaking. Be aware that a mustache or a beard makes speechreading more difficult.

10. When appropriate, include hearing-impaired people in all discussions about them. Hearing-impaired persons sometimes feel quite vulnerable. This approach will aid in alleviating some of those feelings.

11. Ask what you might do to make conversation easier.

12. In larger meetings or any group activity where there is a speaker presenting information, make it mandatory that the speaker use the public address system.

105. What Are Common Emotional Reactions to Hearing Loss?

The initial reaction to having hearing loss can span a range of emotions: shock, denial, depression, sadness, shame, and fear. If a person is born with hearing loss or acquires it during childhood, the teenage years can be extremely stressful and the anger that results from the teasing or rejection of peers can be significant and leave emotional scars. Hearing loss that occurs later in life can impact on a person's feelings of self-worth.

A hearing loss may make you feel depressed and lonely. It may exaggerate your natural tendencies toward being an extrovert or an introvert. Some people with hearing loss may try to monopolize the conversation so they won't need to hear, and others will choose to withdraw so they won't have to strain to hear. You may sometimes become suspicious that others are talking about you if you cannot hear some conversations; that is not an unusual reaction. Some people feel ashamed or embarrassed that they cannot hear.

Because it is more work for you to hear and communicate, you may find that you get very stressed and weary after a day of many interactions. Realizing that these emotional reactions are common among people who experience hearing loss can be the first step to accepting the situation and then finding coping strategies to help you.

106. Are There Support Groups?

The following list of organizations can provide information, assistance, and support. Also see the listing of SHHH affiliates in Appendix 4.

SELF HELP FOR HARD OF HEARING PEOPLE, INC.
(SHHH)
7910 Woodmont Avenue, Suite 1200
Bethesda, MD 20814
(301) 657-2248 (voice)
(301) 657-2249 (TTY)

NATIONAL ASSOCIATION OF THE DEAF
814 Thayer Avenue
Silver Spring, MD 20910
(301) 587-1788 (voice/TTY/TDD)

AMERICAN TINNITUS ASSOCIATION (ATA)
PO Box 5
Portland, OR 97207-0005
(513) 248-9985 (voice)

THE MENIERE'S NETWORK
2000 Church Street, Box 111
Nashville, TN 37236
(800) 545-HEAR (out-of-state)
(615) 329-7807 (instate)

107. What Other Organizations Provide Help?

ACADEMY OF DISPENSING AUDIOLOGISTS
3008 Millwood Avenue
Columbia, SC 29205
(803) 252-5646 (voice)

ACADEMY OF REHABILITATIVE AUDIOLOGY
PO Box 26532
Minneapolis, MN 55426
(612) 920-6098 (voice)

ALEXANDER GRAHAM BELL ASSOCIATION
FOR THE DEAF
3417 Volta Place NW
Washington, DC 20007
(202) 337-5220 (voice)

AMERICAN ACADEMY OF AUDIOLOGY
8201 Greensboro Drive, Suite 300
McLean, VA 22102
(800) AAA-2336 (voice)

AMERICAN ACADEMY OF OTOLARYNGOLOGY—HEAD
AND NECK SURGERY
One Prince Street
Alexandria, VA 22314
(703) 836-4444 (voice)
(703) 683-5100 (fax)

AMERICAN AUDITORY SOCIETY
512 East Canterbury Lane
Phoenix, AZ 85022
(602) 942-4939 (voice)

AMERICAN SPEECH LANGUAGE HEARING ASSOCIATION
10801 Rockville Pike
Rockville, MD 20852
(301) 897-5700 (instate)
(800) 638-6255 (out-of-state)

ASSOCIATION OF LATE-DEAFENED ADULTS
10310 Main Street, Box 274
Fairfax, VA 22030

BETTER HEARING INSTITUTE
5021 B Backlick Road
Annandale, VA 22003
(800) Ear-Well (voice)

BOYS TOWN NATIONAL INSTITUTE FOR
COMMUNICATION DISORDERS IN CHILDREN
Hereditary Hearing Impairment Registry
555 North 30th Street
Omaha, NE 68131
(800) 320-1171 (voice/TTY)

CAPTION CENTER
125 Western Avenue
Boston, MA 02134
(617) 492-9225 (voice/TTY)

MODERN TALKING PICTURE SERVICE, INC.
5000 Park Street North
St. Petersburg, FL 33709
(800) 237-6213 (voice/TTY)
(813) 546-0681 (fax)

COCHLEAR IMPLANT CLUB INTERNATIONAL
PO Box 464
Buffalo, NY 14223
(716) 838-4662 (voice/TTY)

DEAFNESS RESEARCH FOUNDATION
9 E. 38th Street, 7th Floor
New York, NY 10016-0003
(212) 684-6556 (voice/TTY)
(800) 535-3323 (voice only)

GALLAUDET UNIVERSITY
800 Florida Avenue, NE
Washington, DC 20002
(202) 651-5000 (voice)

HEARING EDUCATION AND AWARENESS FOR ROCKERS
(H.E.A.R)
PO Box 460847
San Francisco, CA 94146
(415) 773-9590 (voice)

HEARING INDUSTRIES ASSOCIATION
515 King Street, Suite 420
Alexandria, VA 22314
(703) 684-5744 (voice)

INTERNATIONAL CENTER FOR THE DISABLED
Education & Training Department
340 E. 24th Street
New York, NY 10010
(212) 679-0100 x289 (voice)

INTERNATIONAL CONGRESS OF THE HARD OF HEARING
8203 Lillystone Drive
Bethesda, MD 20817
(301) 365-3548 (voice)

NATIONAL BOARD FOR CERTIFICATION IN HEARING
INSTRUMENT SCIENCES
20361 Middlebelt Road
Livonia, MI 48152
(800) 521-5247 (voice)

NATIONAL CAPTIONING INSTITUTE
1900 Gallows Road Suite 3000
Vienna, VA 22182
(703) 998-2400 (voice/TTY)
(800) 533-WORD (voice)
(800) 321-TDDS (TTY)

NATIONAL ASSOCIATION OF THE DEAF
814 Thayer Avenue
Silver Spring, MD 20910
(301) 587-6282 (voice)
(301) 587-6283 (TTY)

NATIONAL CUED SPEECH ASSOCIATION
1615-B Oberlin Road
PO Box 31345
Raleigh, NC 27622
(919) 828-1218 (voice/TTY)

NATIONAL HEARING AID SOCIETY
20361 Middlebelt Road
Livonia, MI 48152
(313) 478-2610 (voice)

NATIONAL HEARING CONSERVATION ASSOCIATION
611 E. Wells Street
Milwaukee, WI 53202
(414) 276-6045 (voice)

NATIONAL INSTITUTE ON DEAFNESS AND OTHER
COMMUNICATION DISORDERS (NIDCD)
Information Clearinghouse
1 Communication Avenue
Bethesda, MD 20892
(800) 241-1044 (voice)
(800) 241-1055 (TTY)

NATIONAL TECHNICAL INSTITUTE FOR THE DEAF
Rochester Institute of Technology
One Lomb Memorial Drive
PO Box 9887
Rochester, NY 14623-0887
(716) 475-6400 (voice)
(716) 475-2181(TTY)

PAN AMERICAN CONGRESS OF
OTORHINOLARYNGOLOGY—HEAD & NECK SURGERY
University of Miami
School of Medicine
Dept. of Otolaryngology, D-48
PO Box 016960
Miami, FL 33101
(305)549-7995 (voice)
(305) 326-7610 (fax)

PROSPER MENIERE SOCIETY
300 E. Hampden Avenue
Suite 401
Englewood, CO 80110
(303) 850-9545 (voice)

108. What Is ACCESS 2000?

ACCESS 2000: Accessibility for Deaf and Hard of Hearing People is a program designed to promote communication access for persons with hearing impairment. The program has as its objectives:

1. Accessibility for deaf and hard of hearing people in public facilities and service industries

2. Making the International Symbol of Access for Hearing Impairment *(see Figure 5-4)* as familiar as the wheelchair access symbol by the year 2000.

It is a program involving training and education to increase sensitivity to the needs of persons with hearing impairment plus the use of various technical devices to ensure that differing environments will be accessible.

The Northeastern New York ACCESS 2000 Committee, established in May 1988, is sponsored by H.E.A.R. (Hearing Endeavor for the Albany Region), the local chapter of Shhh, Inc. The committee members, who are from various disciplines, meet monthly at The Hearing Center at the Albany Medical Center Hospital in Albany, New York.

The committee has chosen to target the following areas in their focus plan:

1. Health-related facilities, including hospitals and nursing homes

2. Emergency services such as ambulance, police, and fire departments

3. Public gathering places

4. Businesses

5. Government agencies

For further information, contact:

ACCESS 2000, H.E.A.R. CHAPTER OF SHHH
c/o The Hearing Center
Albany Medical Center Hospital
43 New Scotland Avenue
Albany, NY 12208
(518) 262-4535 (voice/TTY)

A list of sample materials from ACCESS 2000 is included in Appendix 6. You may also contact Self Help for Hard of Hearing People, Inc. for more detailed information regarding the Hospital Awareness Program *(see Question 92)*.

Appendices

Glossary

ACOUSTIC NEUROMA A tumor on the auditory nerve.

ACOUSTIC REFLEX The involuntary contraction of the stapedius muscle in the middle ear in response to loud sound. The test for acoustic reflex is one component of the immittance test battery.

ACOUSTIC TRAUMA Damage to the inner ear caused by extremely loud or explosive noise resulting in hearing loss.

AIR BLOWER A rubber bulb that, when squeezed, blows air to dry out a hearing aid or earmold.

AIR CONDUCTION A term usually associated with audiometric testing referring to sound being heard through earphones.

AMERICANS WITH DISABILITIES ACT (ADA) The Americans with Disabilities Act of 1990 Public Law 101-336 prohibits discrimination on the basis of disability by private entities.

AMPLIFIED TELEPHONE A telephone with a built-in amplifier on the handset. Public phones have a volume control button on the wall unit.

ASSISTIVE LISTENING DEVICES AND SYSTEMS (ALDS)
Supplementary systems or devices, other than standard hearing aids, that improve the reception of sound or alert the user to a sound.

AUDIOGRAM A chart showing the results of a hearing evaluation indicating the degree of hearing loss in decibels over a range of specific tones (frequencies). Usually the frequencies from 250 Hz through 8000 Hz are charted on the audiogram.

AUDIOLOGIST A university-trained professional with a master's (MS or MA) or doctorate (PhD or EdD) degree in audiology. The audiologist is responsible for assessing hearing and for providing rehabilitative services to increase the ability of people with hearing loss to function more efficiently in everyday life.

AUDIO LOOP (INDUCTION LOOP) An assistive listening device that uses electromagnetic waves for transmission of sound. The sound from an amplifier is fed into a wire loop worn around the listener's neck or surrounding the seating area that broadcasts to a telecoil that serves as a receiver. Hearing aids with a T-switch can act as a receiver or a special induction receiver can be used to pick up the sound.

AUDIOMETER The electronic instrument used by the audiologist for measuring the threshold of hearing.

AUDIOMETRY Specific procedures by which the threshold of hearing is measured.

AUDITORY BRAINSTEM RESPONSE (ABR) TEST Also called *Brainstem Evoked Response* (BSER), *Brainstem Auditory Evoked Response* (BAER), and *Auditory Evoked Response* (AER), this test objectively measures hearing by placing electrodes on the scalp to record the electrical activity in the brain when sound occurs. It is used for newborn babies, infants, and young children who cannot respond reliably using standard procedures such as visual reinforcement audiometry, play audiometry, or picture identification.

AUDITORY TRAINING EQUIPMENT Supplementary listening systems that increase audibility for the child with hearing loss. The equipment can be a desktop system or an FM listening system.

AURICLE The visible part of the ear, also called the *pinna*.

BASIC HEARING EVALUATION A combination of tests and procedures used by audiologists to measure hearing ability.

BATTERY TESTER A small device that can measure the functional capacity of the hearing aid battery. (A must for caregivers who monitor a hearing aid function for another person.)

BINAURAL Listening with both ears.

BODY HEARING AID A hearing aid in which the microphone, amplifier, and battery are housed in a small unit worn on the body. An earmold is connected to a receiver that is connected by a cord to the hearing aid. This type of hearing aid is capable of providing powerful amplification.

BONE CONDUCTION The process by which sound can be heard from a vibrator placed on the skull, usually behind the ear, which assesses the condition of the nerves of hearing.

BONE CONDUCTION OSCILLATOR A vibrator used for bone conduction audiometry or with some specific types of hearing aids worn by people who, because of ear infections, cannot wear anything in their ear.

CANAL HEARING AIDS Small instruments worn within the ear canal.

CERUMEN Earwax.

CLEAN AID SOLUTION A special solution for sanitizing the earmold and/or hearing aid.

CLOSED CAPTIONS Text display of spoken dialogue and sounds on television and videos visible only to those using a closed caption decoder or a television with a built-in decoder chip.

COCHLEA The snail-like bony cavity that contains the delicate hair cells located in the inner ear. It is about the size of a dried pea.

COMPUTER-ASSISTED NOTE TAKING A visual display, projected on a screen or a monitor, consisting of a summary of the speaker's words that has been typed on a computer keyboard.

CONDUCTIVE HEARING LOSS A hearing loss associated with the functioning of the outer or middle ear.

CUED SPEECH A system of hand shapes used to supplement the information received from speechreading (lipreading).

DEAF *Webster's New World Dictionary College Edition* defines deaf as totally or partially unable to hear. It generally refers to people who usually have little or no useful residual hearing and who employ sign language as their primary mode of communication. Deaf people may also use speechreading, hearing aids, and other assistive technology to aid communication. People who are deaf can be categorized into two groups: *congenitally deaf* (those who were born deaf); and *adventitiously deaf* (those who were born with hearing but whose sense of hearing became nonfunctional later in life).

DECIBEL (dB) A unit for measuring the volume of a sound, equal to the logarithm of the ratio of the intensity of the sound to the intensity of an arbitrarily chosen standard sound.

DEHUMIDIFYING/DRYING KIT A plastic bag or small plastic container with a metal disc filled with silica gel to dry out the hearing aid.

DIGITAL HEARING AIDS Hearing instruments that process sound by converting its wave forms into sequences of binary numbers or digits, processing these sequences and reconverting them into analog electrical waves to generate sounds.

DISPENSING AUDIOLOGIST An audiologist who, in addition to evaluating a person's hearing ability, selects and fits hearing aids; orders the instruments; sells them to the patient; and provides follow-up care.

EARMOLD A specially molded piece of lucite or vinyl material that is attached to a hearing aid to conduct sound into the ear.

ELECTRONYSTAGMOGRAPHY (ENG) A battery of tests that examine eye movements to evaluate the function of the vestibular (balance) system, the hearing mechanism.

ENT CLINIC An abbreviation for *ear, nose, and throat clinic,* a place where hearing loss and problems of the ear are diagnosed and treated.

EUSTACHIAN TUBES The soft tubes connecting the middle ear and the back of the mouth that serve to equalize air pressure and to drain fluids.

FEEDBACK A term that describes what occurs when too much amplified sound escapes from the ear and is picked up by the microphone of the hearing aid, causing a high-pitched whistling sound. The whistling persists until the amplification of the hearing aid is reduced by turning down the gain control. Feedback may occur if the hearing aid or earmold is not properly fit into the ear, if the volume of the hearing aid is set too high, or if an object (e.g., a hat or a hand) comes in contact with the microphone.

FM SYSTEM A transmitter that broadcasts a signal by radio waves from the sound source to a receiver worn by the listener. It is wireless and is useful in large indoor or outdoor areas since the signal can pass through physical obstructions and has a range of several hundred feet.

FREQUENCY The number of sound vibrations per second, expressed in Hertz (Hz), corresponding to the pitch of sound.

HARD OF HEARING The term used to describe a degree of hearing loss ranging from mild to profound for which a person usually receives some benefit from amplification. Most people who are hard of hearing are oralists (communicate by using their voice), although a small number learn sign language. Usually they participate in society by using their residual hearing with hearing aids, speechreading, and assistive devices to facilitate communication.

HEARING AID An instrument that amplifies sound to assist persons with hearing loss. They are distinguished by where they are worn: in the ear (ITE), in the canal (ITC), completely in the canal (CIC), behind the ear (BTE), or on the body.

HEARING AID DEALER A hearing aid salesperson licensed by the state to provide a retail outlet for hearing aids. A hearing aid dealer may use the term *hearing aid specialist* but may not be referred to as an audiologist and is not trained to provide audiological services.

HEARING LOSS The difference between the level of sound that can just be heard by an individual with impaired hearing and a standard level that has been determined by averaging measurements from a group of young hearing people. It is usually expressed in decibels.

HERTZ (Hz) Denotes the pitch or frequency of a sound in cycles per second.

INDUCTION LOOP An induction loop is often in the form of a wire, run around the perimeter of a room or area, that is fed by an amplifier with an electric current. This current produces a magnetic field that can then be picked up by a power loop receiver or by a coil of wire in a hearing aid (selected by moving the switch to "T") and heard as sound by the user.

INFRARED SYSTEM An assistive listening device similar to FM except that it uses invisible light waves to transmit sound. It is often used in theaters.

INNER EAR That part of the ear, particularly the cochlea, that converts mechanical vibrations (sound) into neural messages that are sent to the brain.

INTERNATIONAL SYMBOL OF ACCESS FOR HEARING LOSS The symbol used to denote communication access for people who are hard of hearing or deaf *(see Figure 5-4)*.

INTERPRETER (ORAL) An interpreter who silently mouths the words of the speaker so they are visible on the lips. Used when speechreading is being used to understand the conversation.

INTERPRETER (SIGN LANGUAGE) An interpreter who uses visible movements of the hands, body, and face to replace the vocal elements of spoken language, using the unique grammar of American Sign Language (ASL) or some variety of Sign that uses English and ASL.

IN-THE-EAR HEARING AID A small instrument that is worn entirely within the concha of the outer ear, inserting a short way into the ear canal.

LIPREADING The ability to gain understanding of what is being said by watching the lips as well as by watching the face, expressions, and gestures. The term *speechreading* is now recognized as more descriptive because it includes watching the facial expressions, gestures, and body language as well as the lips.

LOUDNESS DISCOMFORT LEVEL The level of sound that the listener finds uncomfortable to listen to for any period of time.

MASKER A device worn behind the ear or in the ear that produces a rushing noise that may help reduce (mask) head noises (tinnitus).

MASKING During a hearing test, a noise may be presented to one ear to prevent it from picking up sounds presented to the ear that is being tested.

MEDICAL CLEARANCE A required recommendation stating a physician's approval for the purchase of hearing aids, implying that there are no medical contraindications for hearing aid use.

MIDDLE EAR That part of the ear that conducts sound to the inner ear, consisting of the eardrum (tympanic membrane), middle ear bones (ossicle), and the cavity containing them.

MOISTURE GUARD A thin roll of plastic wrap that can be wound around a behind-the-ear hearing aid to protect it from perspiration.

NOTE TAKER A person who takes notes in a notebook, on a blackboard, or on an overhead projector using key words and phrases to enhance the understanding of the person with hearing loss.

OTOACOUSTIC EMISSIONS Very soft sounds generated in the inner ear and detected in the middle ear in a normally functioning ear.

OTOLARYNGOLOGIST A physician (MD or DO) knowledgeable in diseases of the ear, nose, and throat (ENT).

OTOLOGIST A physician who is trained in otolaryngology (the ear, nose, and throat) and who has specialized in problems of the ear.

OTOSCLEROSIS A condition in which the bones of the middle ear become immobile because of bony growth.

OTOSCOPIC EXAMINATION With the use of an otoscope, an instrument with a light and a magnifying glass, the appearance of the outer ear, ear canal, and eardrum is checked for any blockage, inflammation, or infection.

OTOTOXINS Medications or drugs that can damage hearing.

POSTAURICULAR An expression used to describe hearing aids worn behind the ear.

PRELINGUAL HEARING IMPAIRMENT Hearing impairment occurring before speech and language has developed normally in a child.

PRESBYACUSIS Hearing loss associated with living longer.

PURE TONE A sound occurring at one frequency used in audiometry.

PURE TONE AVERAGE An average of hearing thresholds for selected frequencies, usually 500 Hz, 1000 Hz, and 2000 Hz used to express the degree of hearing loss.

REAL EAR MEASUREMENT A method of measuring the amount of amplification from a hearing aid in the user's ear.

RECRUITMENT An abnormally rapid growth of loudness when sound intensity is increased in damaged ears.

RELAY SERVICE Enables text telephone (TTY) users to communicate with non-TTY users by way of a relay service communications operator. The ADA mandated a nationwide relay service to be completed in 1993.

SEMICIRCULAR CANALS The organ of balance connected directly to the cochlea in the inner ear.

SENSORI-NEURAL HEARING LOSS A hearing loss that results from some damage to the inner ear or pathways to the brain, often resulting in distortion of speech sound. This is not usually alleviated by surgical or medical means.

SIGNAGE FOR HEARING ACCESS

| COMMUNICATION ACCESS | TELEPHONE AMPLIFIER | INTERNATIONAL TTY |

SPEECH AUDIOMETRY Testing hearing by using speech, usually lists of isolated words or sentences.

SPEECHREADING See *Lipreading.*

SPEECH RECEPTION TEST (SRT) Using two-syllable words called *spondees* (e.g., *airplane, baseball, rainbow*), the audiologist will ask you to repeat each word heard as the loudness is diminished. Some words are very soft and guessing is allowed. The purpose of the test is a cross-check for the accuracy of the pure tone test results and to check your ability to recognize and repeat words accurately.

SPEECH RECOGNITION TEST Also called a *speech discrimination test,* one-syllable words (e.g., *gun, dog, love*) are presented at a comfortable loudness level based on the speech reception threshold results, and you are asked to repeat the words heard as clearly as you can. This test indicates how clearly you can recognize words and understand them.

T-COIL The part of a hearing aid that picks up magnetic forces generated by an audio loop or specific telephone amplifiers and then converts these forces to normal sounds. It is activated by the telecoil-switch (T-switch).

TEMPORARY THRESHOLD SHIFT (TTS) A loss of hearing associated with the effect of loud noise, which disappears after a period of recovery.

TEXT TELEPHONE (TTY) A communication aid to help people use the telephone by typing their message and receiving it in print. A text telephone must interact with another text telephone or computer. It is also called a TDD.

THRESHOLD OF HEARING The faintest sound that can be consistently heard at each of the tested frequencies in an audiometric evaluation.

TINNITUS Noises in the head or ears.

TYMPANIC MEMBRANE Another name for the eardrum.

TYMPANOGRAM The graph that results from tympanometry, describing the acoustic evaluation of the outer and middle ear's ability to accept and conduct sound.

TYMPANOMETRY The measurement of the outer and middle ear's ability to accept and conduct sound.

UNCOMFORTABLE LOUDNESS LEVEL (ULL) The hearing level at which a listener signals that sound is too loud and not comfortable.

VIDEO TEXT DISPLAY A real-time speech-to-text system in which the words of the speaker are typed on a keyboard similar to the one used by court reporters. The text is projected onto a screen to be read by the audience.

VISUAL ALARM SIGNAL A visual signal that gives notice that an audible event (e.g., a doorbell, a ringing telephone, a crying baby, or a fire alarm) is taking place.

VISUAL REINFORCEMENT AUDIOMETRY (VRA) A lighted or animated toy is used to reward a correct response when testing the hearing of very young children (about two years and younger). When the toy is used to get the child to turn toward the source of the sound, it is called *Conditioned Orientation Response* (COR). The results of the child's responses can be plotted on an audiogram in the same manner as when adults raise their hand, use the signal button, or say yes.

WAX LOOP REMOVER A small plastic piece with a metal point to be used for cleaning cerumen (ear wax) from the nib of the in-the-ear hearing aid or earmold.

APPENDIX TWO

Recommended Readings

Alpiner, J. G., and McCarthy, P. *Rehabilitative Audiology.* Baltimore: Williams and Wilkins, 1987.

Dugan, M. *Keys to Living With Hearing Loss.* New York: Barron's Educational Services, 1997.

Helleberg, M. M. *Your Hearing Loss: How to Break the Sound Barrier.* Chicago: Nelson-Hall, 1979.

Kaplan, H., Ball, S. and Garretson, C., *Speechreading: A Way to Improve Understanding.* Washington, DC: Gallaudet College Press, 1985.

Pope, A. *Hear: Solutions, Skills and Sources for Hard of Hearing People.* New York: DK Publishing, Inc., 1997.

Sandlin, R.E. *Handbook of Hearing Aid Amplification,* Volumes I and II. Boston: College Hill Press, 1988.

Schow, R. L. and Nerbonne, M. A. *Introduction to Aural Rehabilitation.* Baltimore: University Park Press, 1980.

Wayner, D. S. *The Hearing Aid Handbook: User's Guide for Adults.* Washington, DC: Gallaudet University Press, 1990.

Wayner, D. S. *The Hearing Aid Handbook: User's Guide for Children*. Washington, DC: Gallaudet University Press, 1990.

Wayner, D. S. and Abrahamson, J. *Learning To Hear Again*, Austin, Texas: Hear Again, 1996.

Suppliers of Assistive Listening Devices and Systems

AT&T NATIONAL SPECIAL NEEDS CENTER
2001 Route 46, Suite 310
Parsipanny, NJ 07054
(800) 233-1222 (voice)
(800) 833-3232 (TTY)

GENERAL TECHNOLOGIES
7415 Winding Way
Fair Oaks, CA 95628
(800) 328-6684 (voice/TTY)

HARC MERCANTILE LTD.
PO Box 3055
3130 Portage Road
Kalamazoo, MI 49003
(800) 445-9968 (voice)

HARRIS COMMUNICATIONS
15159 Technology Drive
Eden Prairie, MN 55344
(800) 825-6758 (voice)

HITEC GROUP INTERNATIONAL, INC.
8160 Madison Avenue
Burr Ridge, IL 60521-5854
(888) 860-6252 (voice/TTY)

MAXI AIDS
42 Executive Boulevard
PO Box 3209
Farmingdale, NY 11735
(800) 522-6294 (voice)

POTOMAC TECHNOLOGY
One Church Street, Suite 402
Rockville, MD 20850-4158
(301) 762-4005 (voice/TTY)

RADIO SHACK (ALSO VISIT YOUR LOCAL STORE)
Selected Products for People With Special Needs
500 One Tandy Center
Fort Worth, TX 76102
(817) 390-3011

WEITBRECHT COMMUNICATIONS, INC
2656 29th Street Suite 205
Santa Monica, CA 90405
(310) 452-8613 (voice)
(310) 452-5460 (TTY)

Self Help for *Hard* of *Hearing, Inc.* *(SHHH) Affiliates*

THERE ARE MORE THAN 250 SHHH affiliates in 49 states across the United States. Many more are in the planning stages. Chapters sponsor monthly meetings that combine speakers and discussion presented in a communicatively accessible setting. If you are interested in contacting the chapter in your area, or if you would be interested in starting a group, contact the Chapter Development office at the SHHH national office at (301) 657-2248 (voice) or (301) 657-2249 (TTY).

ALABAMA
Birmingham
Rocket City

ALASKA
Fairbanks

ARIZONA
Greater Phoenix
Sun City

ARKANSAS
Little Rock

CALIFORNIA
Banning
Barstow
Camarillo
Conejo Valley
Diablo Valley
Escondido
Fresno
La Mesa
Livermore/Pleasanton/
    SanRamon

Long Beach/Lakewood
Los Angeles/Culver City
Napa (North Bay)
Oakland (East Bay)
Orange County
Peninsula
Redding/Anderson
Redlands
Sacramento
San Diego (Sports Arena)
San Diego (Rancho Bernardo)
San Diego (Pacific Beach)
San Fernando Valley
San Francisco
San Jose
Santa Barbara
Santa Maria Area
Solano County
Ukiah
Ventura/Ojai

COLORADO
Boulder
Central Denver

CONNECTICUT
Central Connecticut
East Haven

DELAWARE
Wilmington

FLORIDA
Boca Raton
Bradenton
Clearwater/St. Petersburg

Delray
Fort Myers
Lauderdale Lakes
Miami (Coral Gables)
Naples
North Port/Port Charlotte
Okaloosa
Palm Beaches
Pensacola
Port St. Lucie
Sarasota
Sun City Center
Tampa

GEORGIA
Aiken-Augusta (SC/GA)
Atlanta
Gainsville-Lanier
Rome

HAWAII
Honolulu

IDAHO
Boise
Coeur d'Alene
Moscow

ILLINOIS
Chicago
    Loop
    Northside
    S. Suburban
    W. Suburban
Jacksonville
North Shore

Peoria
Quad Cities (IL/IA)
Springfield

INDIANA
Evansville
Granger
South Bend
West Lafayette

IOWA
Des Moines
Iowa City/Cedar Rapids
Quad Cities (IL/IA)

KANSAS
Johnson County
Kansas City (KS/MO)

KENTUCKY
Kentucky Lake
Louisville
Northern Kentucky

LOUISIANA
Alexandria
New Orleans
Northwest Louisiana

MARYLAND
Annapolis
Bel Air
Greater Baltimore
Montgomery County
Towson

MASSACHUSETTS
Attleboro
Cape Cod
Greater Boston
Framingham
North of Boston
Plymouth/Duxbury
South Shore
Springfield
Worcester

MICHIGAN
Birmingham
Gaastra
Grand Rapids
Jackson
Kalamazoo
Lansing
Muskegon
Traverse City
Washtenaw Area

MINNESOTA
Central Minnesota
   (St. Cloud)
Minneapolis
Southern Minnesota
   (Fairbault)

MISSISSIPPI
Biloxi
Jackson

MISSOURI
Kansas City (KS/MO)
Lee's Summit

St. Joseph
St. Louis

MONTANA
Billings
Bozeman

NEBRASKA
North Platte
Omaha

NEVADA
Las Vegas

NEW HAMPSHIRE
Manchester/Concord/Nashua

NEW JERSEY
Bergen County
Central Jersey
Madison
Middlesex County
Northwest NJ (Long Valley)
South Jersey

NEW MEXICO
Albuquerque
Roswell
Santa Fe

NEW YORK
Albany
Corning
Finger Lakes
Jamestown
New York City
　　Brooklyn
　　Huntington

Manhattan
North Shore (Roslyn)
South Nassau (Oceanside)
Poughkeepsie
Rochester (Day & Evening)
Syracuse
Utica
Westchester
Western NY (Buffalo)

NORTH CAROLINA
Chapel Hill
Charlotte
Durham
Greensboro
Hendersonville
Raleigh
Wilmington
Winston-Salem

OHIO
Canton Area
Cincinnati
Cleveland Metro
Cleveland West (Rocky River)
Columbus
Lebanon
Lima
Lorain County (Elyria)
Marion
Zanesville

OKLAHOMA
Oklahoma City (Day &
　　Evening)

OREGON

Douglas County
Lane County (Eugene)
Lowestin (Lake Oswego)
Medford
Portland

PENNSYLVANIA

Berks County
Delaware County
    (Springfield)
Grove City
Harrisburg
Lancaster
Lebanon County (Cornwall)
Lehigh Valley
Montgomery County
Philadelphia #1
Philadelphia (Center City)
Pittsburgh
Schuykill County
Squirrel Hill
Wyoming Valley
York Area

RHODE ISLAND

Narragansett
Providence

SOUTH CAROLINA

Aiken-Augusta (SC/GA)
Columbia

SOUTH DAKOTA

Sioux Falls

TENNESSEE

Chattanooga
Knoxville (East Tennessee)
Knoxville (Maryville)
Memphis

TEXAS

Amarillo
Austin
Corpus Christi
Dallas
East Texas (Longview)
El Paso
Fort Worth
Houston
San Antonio

UTAH

Salt Lake City Area

VERMONT

Burlington
Montpelier
Rutland

VIRGINIA

Fredericksburg
Northern Virginia
Roanoke
Sterling/Leesburg
Williamsburg
Winchester

WASHINGTON

Edmonds
Everett
Everson

Horizon House (Seattle)
Lacey
Lake Washington
Port Angeles
Seattle Hear Here
Sedro Woley
South King County
Tacoma
West Seattle

WISCONSIN
Appleton
Fond du Lac
Madison Area
Milwaukee Metro
Minocqua
Stevens Point
Waukesha
Whitewater

WYOMING
Casper

Telecommunications
Relay Service Listings

TTY=telecommunication type-
writer or TDD telecommu-
nication device for the deaf

V=voice

SP=speech

ASCII=computer access

A=computer access

TELEB=telebraille device

ALABAMA
AT&T (Must be billed to an
Alabama exchange)
(800) 548-2546/TTY
(800) 548-2547/V

ALASKA
GCI & Relay Alaska
(800) 770-8973/TTY
(800) 770-8255/V

ARIZONA
MCI/VCD
(800) 367-8939/TTY
(800) 842-4681/V

ARKANSAS
MCI
(800) 285-1131/TTY
(800) 285-1121/V

CALIFORNIA
MCI
(800) 735-2929/TTY
(800) 735-2922/V
(800) 855-3000/SP
(800) 735-0091/ASCII

Sprint (Speech-to-Speech)
(800) 854-7784

COLORADO
Sprint
(800) 659-2656/TTY
(800) 659-3656/V
(800) 659-4656/ASCII

CONNECTICUT
Sprint
(800) 842-9710/TTY
(800) 833-8134/V

DELAWARE
AT&T
(800) 232-5460/TTY
(800) 232-5470/V

DC
AT&T (call must originate in
    the DC area)
(202) 855-1234/TTY
(202) 855-1000/V

FLORIDA
MCI
(800) 955-8771/TTY
(800) 955-8770/V

GEORGIA
AT&T
(800) 255-0056/TTY
(800) 255-0135/V

HAWAII
GTE
(800) 877-8973/TTY/V/A

IDAHO
Hamilton Telephone
(800) 377-3529/TTY
(800) 377-1363/V

ILLINOIS
AT&T
(800) 526-0844/TTY
(800) 526-0857/V
(800) 501-0864/TTY
(Spanish)
(800) 501-0865/V (Spanish)

INDIANA
Sprint
(800) 743-3333/TTY/V/A

IOWA
Sprint
(800) 735-2942/TTY/A
(800) 735-2943/V

KANSAS
Southwestern Bell
(800) 766-3777/TTY/V/A

KENTUCKY
AT&T
(800) 648-6056/TTY
(800) 648-6057/V

LOUISIANA
MCI
(800) 846-5277/TTY
(800) 947-5277/V

MAINE
AT&T
(800) 437-1220/TTY
(207) 955-3323/TTY (instate)
(800) 457-1220/V
207-955-3777/V

MARYLAND
Sprint
(800) 735-2258/TTY/V
(900) 386-3323/TTY

MASSACHUSETTS
MCI
(800) 439-2370/TTY
(800) 439-0183/V

MICHIGAN
Ameritech (Calls must origi-
    nate instate)
(800) 649-3777/TTY/V/A

MINNESOTA
Sprint
(800) 627-3529/TTY/V/A

MISSISSIPPI
AT&T
(800) 582-2233/TTY
(800) 855-1000/V

MISSOURI
Sprint
(800) 735-2966/TTY/A
(800) 735-2466/V

MONTANA
Sprint
(800) 253-4091/TTY/A
(800) 253-4093/V

NEBRASKA
Hamilton Telephone
(800) 833-7352/TTY
(800) 833-0920/V

NEVADA
Sprint
(800) 326-6868/TTY/A
(800) 326-6888/V

NEW HAMPSHIRE
Sprint
(800) 735-2964/TTY/V/A

NEW JERSEY
AT&T
(800) 852-7899/TTY
(800) 852-7897/V

NEW MEXICO
Sprint/NM Relay Network
(800) 659-8331/TTY/A
(800) 659-1779/V

NEW YORK
AT&T
(800) 662-1220/TTY
(800) 421-1220/V

NORTH CAROLINA
MCI
(800) 735-2962/TTY
(800) 735-8262/V

NORTH DAKOTA
Sprint
(800) 366-6888/TTY/A
(800) 366-6889/V

OHIO
Ameritech (Calls must originate instate)
(800) 750-0750/TTY/V/A

OKLAHOMA
Sprint
(800) 722-0353/TTY
(800) 522-8506/V

OREGON
Sprint
(800) 735-2900/TTY
(800) 735-1232/V
(800) 735-0644/ASCII
(800) 735-3896/TTY/V/SP

PENNSYLVANIA
AT&T
(800) 654-5984/TTY
(800) 654-5988/V

PUERTO RICO
AT&T (Voice calls must originate in PR)
(800) 240-2050/TTY
(800) 260-2050/V

Long Distance Calls
(800) 208-2828/TTY

RHODE ISLAND
AT&T
(800) 745-5555/TTY
(800) 745-6575/V
(800) 745-1570/ASCII

SOUTH CAROLINA
Sprint
(800) 735-2905/TTY/V/A

SOUTH DAKOTA
Sprint
(800) 877-1113/TTY/V/A

TENNESSEE
AT&T
(800) 848-0298/TTY
(800) 848-0299/V

TEXAS
Sprint
(800) 735-2989/TTY
(800) 735-2988/V
(800) 735-2991/ASCII

UTAH
Utah Telephone (Calls must originate instate)
Utah Association for the Deaf:
(800) 346-4128/TTY/V
Salt Lake: (801) 298-9484/TTY
Ogden: (801) 546-2982/TTY
Logan: (801) 752-9596/TTY
Provo-Orem: (801) 374-2504/TTY

VERMONT
AT&T (Must be billed to an
    instate exchange)
(800) 253-0191/TTY
(800) 253-0195/V

VIRGINIA
AT&T (Must be billed to an
    instate exchange)
(800) 828-1120/TTY
(800) 828-1140/V

VIRGIN ISLANDS
AT&T (Calls must originate
    within the Virgin Islands)
(800) 440-8477/TTY
(800) 809-8744/V

WASHINGTON
AT&T
(800) 833-6388/TTY
(800) 833-6384/V
(800) 833-6385/TELEB

WEST VIRGINIA
AT&T (Must be billed to an
    instate exchange)
(800) 982-8771/TTY
(800) 982-8772/V

WISCONSIN
MCI
(800) 947-3529/TTY/V
(800) 272-1773/ASCII

WYOMING
Sprint
(800) 877-9965/V
(800) 877-9975/T/A
(900) 463-3323/TTY

SPRINT NATIONAL RELAY
(800) 877-8973/TTY/V/A

MCI NATIONAL RELAY
(800) 688-4889/TTY
(800) 947-8642/V

AT&T NATIONAL RELAY
(800) 855-2880/TTY
(800) 855-2881/V
(800) 855-2882/ASCII
(800) 855-2883/TELEB

FEDERAL INFORMATION
RELAY SERVICE
Sprint
(800) 877-8339/TTY/V

OPERATOR ASSISTANCE FOR
THE DEAF
Sprint
(800) 855-4000/TTY
MCI
(800) 688-4486/TTY
AT&T
(800) 855-1154/TTY

ACCESS 2000

Accessibility for Deaf and
Hard of Hearing People by the Year 2000

Program for Health-Related Facilities

What Is ACCESS 2000?

ACCESS 2000 is a national program to promote communications access for persons with hearing impairment. It has as its objectives:

1. Community-wide accessibility for deaf and hard of hearing people in public facilities and service industries by the year 2000, and

2. Making the International Symbol of Access for hearing impairment *(see Figure 5-4)* as familiar as the "wheelchair" access symbol.

It involves an organized program of training and education to increase sensitivity to the needs of persons with hearing impairment plus the use of different types of assistive, technical devices in order to ensure that various environments will be accessible.

Self Help for Hard of Hearing people (SHHH), a national consumer-based organization, is promoting this program in the United States. Similar programs exist in Canada and Great

Britain. In the northeastern New York region, ACCESS 2000 is sponsored by H.E.A.R., Hearing Endeavor for the Albany Region, a chapter of SHHH.

The ACCESS 2000 Committee of Northeastern New York has chosen to target the following areas in their focus plan:

1. Health-related facilities to include hospitals and nursing homes

2. Emergency services such as ambulance, police, and fire departments

3. Public gathering places: e.g., churches, theaters, etc.

4. Businesses

5. Government agencies

What Are the Goals of ACCESS 2000 in a Medical Facility?

The purpose of ACCESS 2000 is to make the hospital or medical facility more accessible to persons with hearing handicap and to reduce the anxiety and frustration that so often accompany a trip to a medical facility. Better interpersonal communication between the staff and the patient is the thrust of the program. This goal is achieved by:

1. Identification of the patient with hearing impairment. The International Symbol of Access for hearing impairment will be used to identify patients. The symbol will be displayed above the bed, on the front of the chart, on the wristband, and beside the call button at the nursing station. Patients would be prompted (through the use of tabletop tent cards) to identify themselves when they are admitted to a health facility.

2. Instruction of staff regarding the ACCESS 2000 Program and use of good communication strategies. All staff who come in contact with patients or with the public will be informed about the program. They will be trained to help identify patients with hear-

ing loss and will be given specific suggestions on how to communicate with a person with hearing impairment.

Why Do We Need ACCESS 2000 in a Medical Facility?

People who have a hearing loss are not easily identified. Their hearing loss does not show. Sometimes people can have a hearing loss and not be aware of it, even though people around them are. It is even more difficult for people with a hearing impairment to hear when they are not feeling well. When people go into the hospital or to another type of health facility, it is important for them to understand what is happening around them and to feel comfortable. The goal of implementing this program in a health-related facility is to ensure accessibility to medical services for persons with hearing impairment, to create a supportive communication environment, and to avoid potentially dangerous miscommunications.

How Can the Program Be Implemented?

The program starts at the door of the facility, where the International Symbol of Access for hearing impairment is prominently displayed. The ACCESS 2000 symbol is also displayed at various intake stations. One side of the display faces the patient and reads: "Tell us if you have a hearing problem. It helps!" The other side of the display, which faces the staff person, contains some rules of good communication. Throughout the hospital—at the nurses' stations, doctors' lounges, waiting rooms, admissions areas, and in the administration areas—are flyers and cards displaying the International Symbol of Access for hearing impairment and the accompanying rules for good communication. Instructional sessions are scheduled on a recurring basis for the nurses, physicians, administrative personnel, and any staff who have contact with the public.

What Are the Potential Services to Be Targeted?

Each health-related facility will have its own priorities regarding who needs to be instructed about ACCESS 2000. Potential target staff might include: physicians, nursing, emergency room, admissions, registration, pharmacy, operating and recovery rooms, patient and family services, transportation, food service, business office, etc. This list should include anyone in a facility who has direct inpatient or outpatient contact, including contact with visitors.

What Materials Will Be Used?

A program should be developed that is tailored to each individual facility. The International Symbol of Access for hearing impairment is the cornerstone of identification for this program, and is available on the following:

- Tent card to be put on tabletops or on counters

- Patient information brochure

- Access symbol sticker for wristband and intercom/call lights

- Large access symbol for over bed, at nursing station, on door, on medical records, or chart cover

- Hearing aid information sheet, if applicable

- Poster with access symbol and communication tips

Assistive Listening Devices (ALDs) and/or systems that may be used in any facility to make it more hearing accessible include:

- Telephone amplifiers

- Personal amplifiers (e.g., Williams Sound "PockeTalkers")

- Telecaptioning decoders

- FM listening systems

- Audio loops

■Infrared systems

■TDD (Telecommunication Device for the Deaf)

■Light signaling devices for the telephone, fire alarms, etc.

For further information about implementation of the ACCESS 2000 Program for Health-Related Facilities write to:

ACCESS 2000/H.E.A.R. CHAPTER OF SHHH
c/o The Hearing Center
43 New Scotland Avenue
Albany, NY 12208
or call: (518) 262-4535 (voice/TTY)

Information about ordering supplies and demonstration of equipment is available at the above address.

ACCESS 2000 Materials

Starter Packet—Includes Program Description (small poster, 4 tent cards, 2 brochures, 10 small Access 2000 stickers, 1 larger symbol sticker, 2 Communicards, and Access 2000 "We Listen" buttons

PRICE INCLUDES SHIPPING AND HANDLING	$5.00
Brochure "The Hearing Impaired Patient"	$0.50
Tent Card "Tips" (17" x 4 1/2" unfolded)	$0.30
Tent Card "Tell Us" (5" x 7" unfolded)	$0.20
Access Symbol (1" x 3/4") Roll of 200	$2.50
Access Symbol (1" x 3/4") Roll of 1000	$10.00
Access Symbol "We Listen" Button (1 1/2" x 1 1/2")	$1.00
Access Symbol Dress Pin (5/8" x 5/8") Clasp or Military	$3.00
Personal Communicard "Tips" on back (2 1/8" x 3/8")	$0.30
Brochure "The Patient Wears Hearing Aid"	$0.25
Poster "Tips" (8 1/2" x 11")	$0.25
Program Description Hearing Access 2000	$0.25
Access 2000 Symbol Sticker (4" x 4")	$0.25

SUBTOTAL _____

SHIPPING AND HANDLING
Orders Under $200 include $3.00
Orders Between $201 and $400 include $4.50
Orders Over $401 include $6.00 _____

TOTAL AMOUNT _____

Make checks payable to H.E.A.R. Access 2000

H.E.A.R. ACCESS 2000
c/o The Hearing Center
43 New Scotland Avenue
Albany, NY 12208

The *Five-Minute Hearing Test*

DIRECTIONS: Mark the column that best describes the frequency with which you experience each situation or feeling below.

	Almost Always	*Half the Time*	*Occasionally*	*Never*

1. I have a problem hearing over the telephone.

    ❏   ❏   ❏   ❏

2. I have trouble following the conversation when two or more people are talking at the same time.

    ❏   ❏   ❏   ❏

3. People complain that I turn the TV volume too high.

    ❏   ❏   ❏   ❏

4. I have to strain to understand conversations.

    ❏   ❏   ❏   ❏

5. I miss hearing some common sounds like the phone or doorbell ringing. ❏   ❏   ❏   ❏

6. I have trouble hearing conversations in a noisy background such as a party. ❏   ❏   ❏   ❏

7. I get confused about where sounds come from.

    ❏   ❏   ❏   ❏

8. I misunderstand some words in a sentence and need to ask people to repeat themselves.

    ❏   ❏   ❏   ❏

9. I especially have trouble understanding the speech of women and children. ❑   ❑   ❑   ❑

10. I have worked in noisy environments (assembly lines, jackhammers, jet engines, etc.).
❑   ❑   ❑   ❑

11. I hear fine—if people just speak clearly.
❑   ❑   ❑   ❑

12. People get annoyed because I misunderstand what they say.
❑   ❑   ❑   ❑

13. I misunderstand what others are saying and make inappropriate responses.
❑   ❑   ❑   ❑

14. I avoid social activities because I cannot hear well and fear I'll reply improperly.
❑   ❑   ❑   ❑

15. (To be answered by a family member or friend.) Do you think this person has a hearing loss?
❑   ❑   ❑   ❑

Total answers this column:

_____   _____   _____   _____

Factor: x3   x2   x1   x0

Multiple factor times answers·

_____   _____   _____   _____

If you have relatives with hearing loss, add 3 pts:

GRAND TOTAL: _____

RECOMMENDATIONS: The AAO-HNS recommends these actions for the following scores

0–5 Your hearing is fine. No action required.

6–9 Suggest you see an Ear-Nose-Throat (ENT) physician.

10+ Strongly recommend you see an ENT physician.

Index